Pharmacological and Psychosocial Treatments in Schizophrenia

Cover artwork: 'The Tracksuit' by Tim Cartledge;
private collection of David Castle

Pharmacological and Psychosocial Treatments in Schizophrenia

Edited by

David Castle MSc MD MRCPsych FRANZCP
Professorial Fellow
Mental Health Research Institute
and University of Melbourne
Victoria
Australia

David L Copolov PhD MBBS FRACP FRANZCP
Director/Professor
Mental Health Research Institute of Victoria
Victoria
Australia

Til Wykes Mphil PhD
Professor of Clinical Psychology and Rehabilitation
Head of Centre for Recovery in Severe Psychosis and
Service User Research Enterprise
Institute of Psychiatry
London
UK

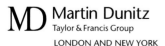

Martin Dunitz
Taylor & Francis Group
LONDON AND NEW YORK

© 2003 Martin Dunitz Ltd, a member of the Taylor & Francis Group

First published in the United Kingdom in 2003
By Martin Dunitz, Taylor & Francis Group plc, 11 New Fetter Lane, London EC4P 4EE

Tel.: +44 (0) 20 7483 9855
Fax.: +44 (0) 20 7842 2298
E-mail: info@dunitz.co.uk
Website: http://www.dunitz.co.uk

Although every effort has been made to ensure that all owners of copyright material have been acknowledged in this publication, we would be glad to acknowledge in subsequent reprints or editions any omissions brought to our attention.

Although every effort has been made to ensure that drug doses and other information are presented accurately in this pubication, the ultimate responsibility rests with the prescribing physician. Neither the publishers nor the authors can be held responsible for errors or for any consequences arising from the use of information contained herein. For detailed prescribing information or instructions on the use of any product or procedure discussed herein, please consult the prescribing information or instructional material issued by the manufacturer.

A CIP record for this book is available from the British Library.

ISBN 1 84184 268 0

Distributed in the USA by
Fulfilment Center
Taylor & Francis
10650 Tobben Drive
Independence, KY 41051, USA
Toll Free Tel: +1 800 634 7064
E-mail: taylorandfrancis@thomsonlearning.com

Distributed in Canada by
Taylor & Francis
74 Rolark Drive
Scarborough, Ontario M1R 4G2, Canada
Toll Free Tel: +1 877 226 2237
E-mail: tal_fran@istar.ca

Distributed in the rest of the World by
Thomson Publishing Services
Cheriton House
North Way
Andover, Hampshire SP10 5BE, UK
Tel: +44 (0)1264 332424
E-mail: salesorder.tandf@thomsonpublishingservices.co.uk

Composition by Wearset Ltd, Boldon, Tyne and Wear

Printed and bound in Great Britain by The Cromwell Press, Trowbridge.

Contents

Contributors

Deirdre Alderton Postgrad Cert Psych Pharm, Postgrad Dip Hosp Pharm
Senior Pharmacist
Fremantle Hospital and Health Service
Fremantle
Western Australia

Christine Barrowclough MSc PhD
Reader in Clinical Psychology, University of Manchester; Honorary
Consultant Clinical Psychologist, Pennine Care Trust;
Academic Division of Clinical Psychology
School of Psychiatry and Behavioural Sciences
Second Floor Education and Research Centre
Wythenshawe Hospital
Manchester
UK

Morris D Bell PhD ABPP
Career Research Scientist for Rehabilitation Research and Development
Service of the Department of Veterans Affairs Health Service; Associate
Professor, Department of Psychiatry, Yale University School of Medicine
West Haven, CT
USA

David Castle MSc MD MRCPsych FRANZCP
Professorial Fellow
Mental Health Research Institute
and University of Melbourne
Victoria, Australia

David L Copolov PhD MBBS FRACP FRANZCP
Director; Professor
Mental Health Research Institute of Victoria
Victoria
Australia

Peter Hayward PhD
Consultant Clinical Psychologist
South London and Maudsley NHS Trust; Honorary Lecturer in
Psychology, Institute of Psychiatry
Kings College
London UK

Wynne James RMN DipN
Dual Diagnosis Liaison Officer
Alma Street Centre
Fremantle Hospital,
Fremantle, Western Australia

Til Wykes MPhil PhD
Professor of Clinical Psychology and Rehabilitation;
Head of the Centre for Recovery in Severe Psychosis and Service User
Research Enterprise
Institute of Psychiatry
London
UK

Foreword

The appearance of this book is a timely reminder of the need for a more holistic approach to the treatment of schizophrenia and in particular puts psychosocial treatments very firmly back onto the agenda. There can be no doubt that a revolution has occurred in the treatment of schizophrenia since the discovery of the first antipsychotic medication, chlorpromazine, in the 1950s. Since then continuing pharmacological progress has been made, bringing schizophrenia into the pantheon of treatable conditions and countering its previous reputation as an inevitably chronic deteriorating illness symbolized by Kraepelin's name for it, 'Dementia Praecox'. In addition, these advances have brought schizophrenia to the attention of multinational pharmaceutical companies intent on improving the drugs available for its treatment. These major changes, possibly the most significant in the history of the treatment of the psychoses over the preceding millennium, have been paralleled by the growth of treatment in the community and the gradual winding down of care in the asylums. But as with most reforms, as the words of a popular song put it, 'something is gained but something is lost'. What has been gained are much more effective biological treatments of the positive, negative, cognitive and mood symptoms of schizophrenia, but what has been lost are the day to day interactions that inevitably occurred between staff looking after patients in asylums, and the structured rehabilitation programmes devised within those hospitals to try to compensate such patients for the deficiencies that the combination of their illness and institutionalization had led to.

Psychosocial treatments for schizophrenia, whilst perhaps not lagging behind, have not received the publicity and attention they deserve, both in their own right and as complementary to psychopharmacological advances. This book highlights the evidence base for such interventions, fragile as it might be in some cases, robust in others. It is a matter of considerable concern that despite this evidence base, only a limited number of these treatments are being offered to a limited number of patients in a limited number of settings around the world. This is one of the major current deficiencies of community psychiatry in relation to the treatment of the severely mentally ill. The only widely used psychosocial interventions remain assessment, monitoring and general support, rather than the application of specific interventions focused on the specific symptoms and disabilities that have arisen both as a direct result of the illness itself, or secondary to the major deficiencies in social support and life skills capacities that can accompany it.

Over the past few years the development of various sets of international guidelines have attempted to overcome this unsatisfactory state of affairs by seeking to place the patient (and their family) once again at the centre of therapeutic endeavours and encouraging mental health professionals to offer the patient and their families a broader therapeutic approach. But the translation of the research evidence into practice is proving a real challenge: overworked, undertrained mental health workers claim not to be able to offer what the literature suggests could be of significant benefit to their patients. This book will go some way in helping to solve that particular problem in that it brings together the relevant literature from several decades in a single volume, offering hope to therapists, patients and families of what can be achieved if psychosocial interventions complement the psychopharmacological treatments that have been progressively available over the second half of the last century. The book is also very practical, providing clear descriptions of what can be offered and how the interventions can be delivered.

I am particularly pleased that two of the editors have professorial appointments in the Department of Psychiatry at The University of Melbourne, being associated with one of our affiliated institutions, the Mental Health Research Institute of Victoria, where Australia's first national Schizophrenia Research Unit was established in the late 1980s under the co-direction of one of the co-editors (Professor Copolov) and myself. I am also pleased that the third co-editor is a member of the Institute of Psychiatry in London, UK, with which our department and the Mental Health Research Institute of Victoria have had such productive relationships over many years, ones which hopefully this book will continue to foster.

I commend this book to all health professionals who work with both patients and their families, who suffer from this most stigmatizing of illnesses.

Professor Bruce Singh
Cato Professor, and Head, Department of Psychiatry,
The University of Melbourne, Australia

Preface

This book aims to provide a succinct clinical overview of key areas pertinent to the holistic treatment of people with schizophrenia. In this context, it is acknowledged that there are a profusion of titles addressing pharmacological aspects of the treatment of schizophrenia and in this book only one of the 10 chapters is devoted to pharmacological treatments, pulling together much of what is current in the literature regarding the newer antipsychotic agents, and providing clinical pointers and guidelines for their use.

The rest of the book deals with psychosocial interventions for specific aspects of schizophrenia symptomatology and disability that have been shown to offer major benefits to recovery in the disorder. Chapters on persistant delusions and hallucinations, negative symptoms, and cognitive disturbance provide brief overviews of the relevant literature, notably on therapeutic interventions, and guidance for clinicians dealing with people with these often distressing and disabling symptoms. The associated and underrecognized problems of anxiety and depression are dealt with separately, as these symptoms are often not adequately addressed in clinical settings; both pharmacological and psychosocial strategies to manage such symptoms are outlined.

Substance abuse is increasingly recognized as a major source of added morbidity in people with schizophrenia. Chapter 6 explores the reasons for the high rates of comorbidity, and outlines approaches to engagement and treatment of such individuals. Chapter 7 discusses the management of acute arousal in schizophrenia – a difficult and potentially traumatic scenario for patients, families and staff alike – and suggestions regarding medications are nested in recommendations regarding a comprehensive and individualized approach to this clinical situation.

Given the all too common problems with engagement in the adherence to treatment by people with schizophrenia, Chapter 8 is devoted to this important topic. It suggests that the building of an alliance of mutual respect and understanding is crucial to successful engagement in the treatment process. The importance of work for people with schizophrenia is outlined in Chapter 9, and strategies that might be effective in assisting patients return to work are considered.

Finally, the family context is addressed, both from the point of view of the patient within a family and the impact an ill loved one has on the family. Again, pertinent treatment interventions are outlined and suggestions are made about how to assist the whole family unit deal with what can be a devastating disorder.

Thus, we have striven to provide clinicians with a succinct, practical guide to the treatment of people with schizophrenia. We have also tried to instil in our readers a real sense of optimism regarding the treatment of this condition: newer and well-validated therapeutic interventions are providing new hope for schizophrenia patients, their families and clinicians.

David Castle, David Copolov, Til Wykes

Disclaimer

Acknowledgements

A number of individuals gave helpful advice regarding various chapters of this book, at varying stages of production. We thank these people, who include Shon Lewis (Manchester, UK), Peter Norrie (Adelaide, Australia), Josh Geffen (Brisbane, Australia), Dan Lubman (Melbourne, Australia), Allan White (Newcastle, Australia), Christine Culhane (Melbourne, Australia), John Farhall (Melbourne, Australia) and John Fielding (Melbourne, Australia). For administrative assistance, we thank, in particular, Silvian van der Merwe. Professor Castle acknowledges with thanks the support of the Harold Mitchell Foundation.

chapter 1

Psychopharmacological management of schizophrenia

David Castle and Deirdre Alderton

It is now well established that antipsychotic medications are one of the mainstays of treatment for psychotic disorders. This has been shown to be the case for both acute management and maintenance treatment aimed at reducing relapse (Kane and Marder, 1993). This chapter concentrates on the pharmacological aspects of the initial and ongoing treatment of psychosis (the management of acute arousal in psychosis is covered in Chapter 7).

Historical background

The discovery of the calming effects of chlorpromazine in the 1950s set the modern pharmacological management of psychotic disorders in motion. Further antipsychotics were soon developed, based on the notion that it was the dopamine D2 blockade in the brain that mediated the antipsychotic effects. Haloperidol was the 'cleanest' D2 blocker of all these earlier agents and became the benchmark against which other agents were measured.

One of the drawbacks of the older, so-called typical antipsychotics is their propensity to produce extrapyramidal side effects (EPSE) such as parkinsonism, dystonias and akathisia, and the longer term problem of tardive dyskinesia (TD) (Jibson and Tandon, 1998) (see Table 1.1). It was thus with great interest that the atypical antipsychotic clozapine was welcomed to the marketplace in the mid-1960s. Clozapine was noted to be a potent antipsychotic with minimal propensity to EPSE/TD and particular efficacy in so-called treatment-resistant cases. However, the limitations of clozapine, notably its propensity to cause a potentially

Table 1.1 Extrapyramidal side effects (EPSE) of antipsychotic drugs

Type of EPSE	Clinical features
Parkinsonism	Mask-like face Muscle rigidity ('cog-wheeling'), shuffling gait (festination, retropulsion) and diminished arm swing 'Pill-rolling' tremor,
Dystonia	**Acute** Involuntary sustained spasm of muscles, notably head and neck (e.g. facial grimacing, protrusion of tongue, opisthotonus, oculogyric crisis); may be painful **Chronic** Sustained involuntary spasm of skeletal muscles, resulting in abnormal posture (e.g. trunk)
Akathisia	**Subjective:** feeling of inner restlessness, with a drive to move **Objective:** frequent changes of posture, inability to sit still, constant walking
Tardive dyskinesia	**Orobuccofaciolingual:** abnormal involuntary movements of face, tongue and lips, with chewing movements, tongue movement, puckering of lips, and grimacing May be associated **truncal** movements and choreoathetoid movements of the **extremities**

fatal agranulocytosis in around 1% of patients, led to its withdrawal in a number of countries in the 1970s (it was reintroduced in the late 1980s, with strict haematological monitoring controls), and the race was on to develop clozapine-like drugs that did not cause blood dyscrasias.

Based on the belief that the atypicality of clozapine was consequent upon its high ratio of serotonin ($5HT_2$):dopamine D2 receptor occupancy, Janssen Pharmaceuticals produced risperidone, which mimicked that particular pharmacological property of clozapine. This product was the first novel atypical antipsychotic to be marketed, and showed a relatively benign side-effect profile compared to haloperidol, though EPSE still occurred at higher doses (see Stahl, 1999). Subsequent novel atypicals include olanzapine, quetiapine, zotepine, sertindole and ziprasidone. Most recently, there have been clinical trials of the partial D2 agonist aripiprazole.

Typical antipsychotics

There are various definitions of typical and atypical antipsychotics. Here, typical antipsychotics are considered to be those drugs that tend (at antipsychotic doses) to produce EPSE. Table 1.2 shows the main typical agents, by class, and their side effects – it should be noted that not all these agents are available in some countries.

The most potent D2 blockers, and notably those without intrinsic anticholinergic properties (i.e. haloperidol), are most likely to cause EPSE, though these effects can occur at higher doses of any of these agents. Other side effects of the typical antipsychotics also tend to be a reflection of receptor binding. For example, those agents with potent H1 blockade tend to be sedating; those with peripheral anticholinergic (muscarinic) effects have a propensity to cause dry mouth, constipation, urinary retention and blurring of vision; and those with alpha-adrenergic blockade can cause problematic postural hypotension. Other potential effects of these agents include weight gain, hyperprolactinaemia (which can result in sexual dysfunction and galactorrhoea), and lowering of the seizure threshold.

Table 1.2 Typical antipsychotics (oral)

Drug	Adult oral maximum dose (mg daily) (BNF)	Half-life (hours)	Anticholinergic	Cardiac	EPSE*	Hypotension	Sedation
Phenothiazines							
Chlorpromazine	1000	16–30	+++	++	++	+++	+++
Levomepromazine (methotrimeprazine)	1000	16–78	+++	++	++	+++	+++
Promazine	800	–	++	++	+	++	++
Thioridazine	600	9–30	++	+++	+	++	++
Pericyazine	300	–	+	++	+	++	+++
Fluphenazine	20	13–58	++	++	+++	+	++
Perphenazine	24	9–21	+	++	+++	+	++
Trifluoperazine	20	13	0	++	+++	+	+
Butyrophenones							
Benperidol	1.5	–	?	?	?	+	++
Haloperidol	30	12–36	+	++	+++	+	+
Droperidol	120	2–4	++	+++	+++	++	++

Table 1.2 continued

Drug	Adult oral maximum dose (mg daily) (BNF)	Half-life (hours)	Anticholinergic	Cardiac	EPSE*	Hypotension	Sedation
Thioxanthines							
Thiothixene	40	34	?	?	?	?	?
Flupenthixol	18	26–36	++	+/–	++	+/–	+
Zuclopenthixol	150	12–28	++	+	+++	+	++
Dibenzoxazepine							
Loxapine	250	8–30	++	+	+++	+	++
Diphenylbutylpiperidine							
Pimozide	20	29–55	+	+++	++	+	+
Substituted benzamides							
Sulpiride	2400	–	+	0	+/–	+/–	+

*Extrapyramidal side-effects.

+++, Marked effect; ++, moderate effect; +, mild effect; +/–, minimal effect at usual therapeutic doses; 0, little or nothing reported; ?, no information available.

BNF, British National Formulary

Adapted from Stephen Bazire (Psychotropic Drug Directory 2001/02, Mark Allen Publishing Ltd, Salisbury, UK, 2002, 138) with permission.

There are other particular side effects of certain agents that might influence prescribing habits [for a comprehensive list of particular side effects see Bezchlibnyk-Butler and Jeffries (2001)]. Of particular concern is the effect some antipsychotics have on cardiac conduction, notably prolongation of the QTc interval, with the potential for sudden death. Pimozide has long been identified in this regard, especially at high doses, and electrocardiogram monitoring is required. More recently, concern about thioridazine has led to restriction of its use in many countries and the oral form of droperidol has been withdrawn, with restrictions placed on the use of the parenteral form, in some countries. Other side effects are less dangerous but also affect prescribing. For example, chlorpromazine results in a photosensitivity that makes its use in sunny climes problematic, while thioridazine at high doses over prolonged usage can result in retinitis pigmentosa.

Atypical antipsychotics

A number of agents have now been developed that demonstrate antipsychotic efficacy at doses that do not usually result in EPSE. These agents are often referred to as either novel or atypical antipsychotics. To avoid confusion with clozapine, which is the archetypal atypical antipsychotic, these agents are referred to here as novel atypicals; when clozapine is grouped with them, they are jointly referred to as atypicals. It should be emphasized, however, that this group contains a number of drug types, with differences in receptor-binding profiles, different side effects and possibly differential efficacies against particular symptoms in different patients. The main current drugs in this group, along with their side effects, are given in Table 1.3; again, not all drugs are available in all countries. Sertindole is not shown, as it has been withdrawn due to concerns regarding effects on cardiac conduction (see Brown et al, 1999). It should be noted that a usual dose range is provided for each agent: this is on the basis of the literature and clinical experience, and does not preclude the use of lower or higher doses in some patients, e.g. low doses are often used in the elderly and higher doses in partial responders. As

Table 1.3 Atypical antipsychotics

DRUG	Usual adult oral daily dose (mg daily)	Half-life (hours)	Anticholinergic	Cardiac	EPSE*	Hypotension	Sedation	Seizure risk	Weight gain	Haematologic	Prolactin elevation
Clozapine[t]	300–500	5–16	+++	+++	0	++	+++	+++[a]	+++	+++	0
Olanzapine[t]	10–20	21–54	+	+	+/–	+/–	++	+	+++	+	+/–
Quetiapine[t]	300–450	6–7	+	+	0	+	++	+	+	+	+/–
Risperidone[t]	2–6	20–24	0	+	+	++	+	+	+	+	+
Zotepine[t]	150–300	?	++	++	+	++	+	+	?	?	?
Amisulpride[§]	400–1200	12	0	+/–	+/–	+/–	+/–	0	+/–	0	+

* Extrapyramidal side effects.

+++, Marked effect (+++[a], dose dependent); ++, moderate effect; +, mild effect; +/–, minimal effect at usual therapeutic doses; 0, little or nothing reported; ?, no information available.

Adapted from: [t]Stephen Bazire (*Psychotropic Drug Directory 2001/02*, Mark Allen Publishing Ltd, Salisbury, UK, 2002, 138) and [‡]Davis R, Markham A (*New Drug Profile: Ziprasidone. CNS Drugs* 1997, 8, 153–162) with permission.
[§] Curran MP, Perry CM. (*Amisulpride: a review of its use in the management of schizophrenia. Drugs* 2001; 61, 2123–2150.)

always, the judgement about dosing is based on clinical response and side-effect burden.

It is still unclear as to which drug would be most beneficial for each individual patient, and often clinical trial and error guides therapeutic interventions. Certainly, efficacy against positive psychotic symptoms seems to be similar between agents; clozapine and possibly quetiapine have some advantage for negative symptoms [see Stahl (1999) and Chapter 3]. It should be noted that amisulpride at low dose (50–300 mg per day) also has benefit for negative symptoms (Leucht et al, 2002). In clinical practice, it is the side-effect profile that probably plays the main part in the determination of drug choice: e.g. sedation and weight gain with olanzapine, the problems of EPSE at high doses, and raised pro-lactin levels with risperidone, and the potential for cardiac conduction problems with ziprasidone might mitigate against the use of each of these agents for particular patients. Stahl (1999) provides useful clinical pearls of wisdom about these agents.

Treatment approaches to early episode psychosis

The atypical antipsychotics have revolutionized the pharmacological management of early episode psychosis and are promoted by most clinicians as the drugs of first choice in such patients. Figure 1.1 shows a treatment algorithm for a patient in their first episode of illness: it should be noted that novel atypical agents are promoted first line and if one atypical fails, or produces intolerable side effects, then a trial of at least one different novel atypical is suggested before reverting to either a typical agent or clozapine. In some countries, notably France, amisulpride is used as a first line for many patients and has a low side effect burden (see Table 1.3). Some clinicians believe that typical agents are more potent than atypicals for some patients and would use these before clozapine; others believe that the particular benefits that can accrue with clozapine treatment should sway clinicians to use this agent earlier in treatment (Taylor et al, 2001).

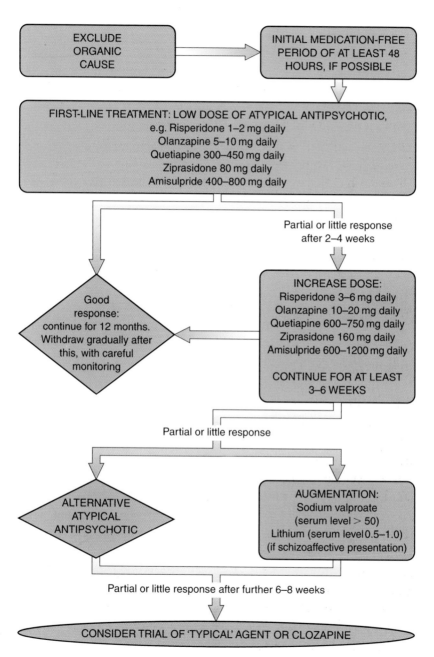

Figure 1.1 *Treatment guidelines: early episode psychosis.*

Treatment of relapse of psychosis

For patients who are established on a typical antipsychotic and who experience a relapse of psychosis, a suggested treatment algorithm is presented in Figure 1.2. The rationale is that if the prior agent was effective and well tolerated, then that agent should be reinstituted. Having said this, some clinicians would consider relapse as an opportunity to change to an atypical antipsychotic. Certainly, if the patient was either inadequately controlled, or experienced EPSE or TD on the typical agent, a change to an atypical should be considered. It is also important to ascertain the cause of the relapse: if it was due to non-adherence to medication, then this would need to be investigated, and if side effects were a contributing factor, this would sway one to change to an atypical antipsychotic.

Treatment resistance and the place of clozapine

In terms of response to medication, the criteria for treatment resistance in schizophrenia usually include at least two failed treatments trials with antipsychotics from at least two different classes (see Lindenmayer, 2000). The domains usually assessed are psychotic symptoms but, given the scope of symptoms and disabilities associated with schizophrenia, it is important to look at the individual in a holistic manner, including associated symptoms such as depression and anxiety, as well as relationships, social and occupational functioning, and overall quality of life. Here, attention is given to the role of medication in treatment resistance. First, the role of clozapine is considered and then pharmacological augmentation strategies. It should be noted that there is some preliminary evidence to suggest that novel atypical antipsychotics will prove beneficial for some treatment-resistant patients, but their precise place in the treatment of such patients is not yet clear (see Meltzer and Fatemi, 1998). The reader is referred to other chapters in this book for broader psychological and social aspects of the treatment of persistent symptoms and disabilities in schizophrenia.

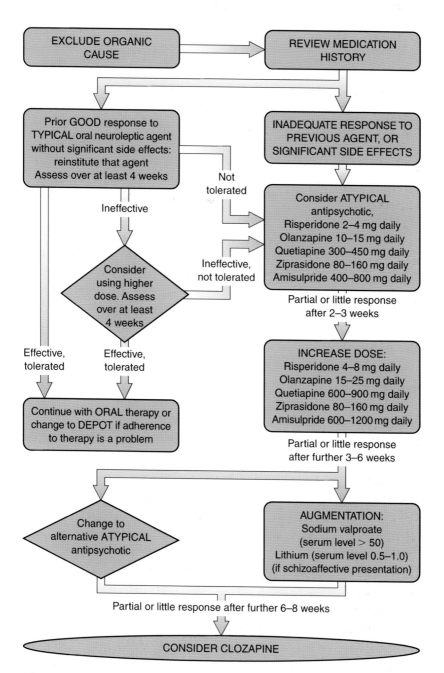

Figure 1.2 *Treatment guidelines: relapse or exacerbation of schizophrenia.*

As discussed above, clozapine was the first atypical antipsychotic in that it does not cause EPSE at therapeutic doses and is associated with an apparent negligible rate of TD. It also appears to have particular benefit in the treatment of patients who have failed to respond to other antipsychotics, i.e. those who are considered to be treatment resistant. There is also some evidence to suggest that clozapine has particular efficacy against the negative symptoms of schizophrenia and might enhance some domains of cognitive function (see Chapters 3 and 4).

Clozapine does, however, produce a number of side effects that limit its use. Most dangerous of these is agranulocytosis, which can be fatal. This potential hazard is addressed by blood monitoring, as outlined in Figure 1.3 (note that monitoring regulations differ between countries, but the principles remain the same). Other side effects include sedation, weight gain, sialorrhoea and lowering of the seizure threshold, which can result in convulsions, expressly at high doses. Hypotension, tachycardia and cardiac conduction abnormalities can also occur (Wagstaff and Bryson, 1995). There is also a risk, albeit low, of potentially fatal cardiomyopathy (Kilian et al, 1999), for which some centres have introduced regular cardiac monitoring for patients on clozapine.

Furthermore, patients who discontinue clozapine abruptly often experience a withdrawal reaction, in part mediated by cholinergic rebound (Wagstaff and Bryson, 1995). There is also clinical evidence that

---

Figure 1.3 Flow chart for treatment commencement and maintenance on clozapine – Australian protocol. WBC, Total white blood cell count; NC, neutrophil cell count; CAP, Clozapine Alert Program (FH Faulding); CPMS, Clozaril Patient Monitoring System (Novartis). Notes for the use of clozapine: (a) all patients must be registered with either the CAP or the CPMS national database; (b) all patients must have blood tests at least weekly for 18 weeks and at least every 4 weeks thereafter; (c) extra blood tests, immediately and twice weekly, are required if symptoms of infection are observed, e.g. sore throat and mouth ulcers; (d) if treatment is stopped for non-haematological reasons then patients on weekly monitoring should continue blood monitoring at least weekly for 4 weeks, patients on weekly monitoring should have one further blood count 4 weeks after ceasing treatment; (e) only medical officers and pharmacists registered with the CAP or the CPMS databases may prescribe and dispense clozapine. Further information can be obtained from the CAP and CPMS protocols, which may vary in different countries, so the relevant national clozapine registration centre should be consulted prior to prescribing.

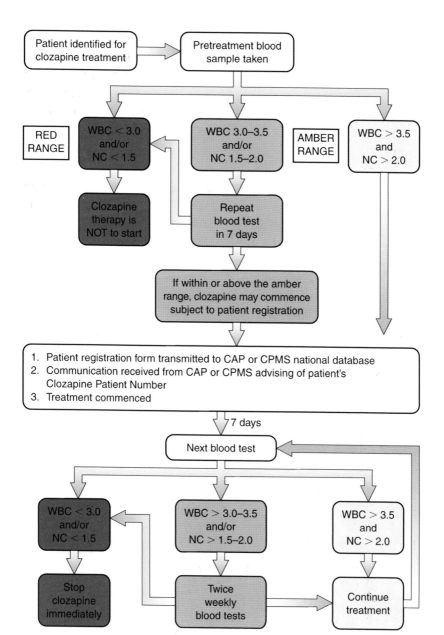

once patients have discontinued clozapine and relapsed, then their chance of responding to rechallenge with clozapine is reduced. Because of these factors, patients on clozapine should be accepting of treatment and close cooperation with the treating team is important. In cases where there is an inadequate response to clozapine, a number of augmentation strategies might be considered (see below).

Augmentation strategies

Another approach to treatment resistance is augmentation with another psychotropic agent. Whilst often applied in clinical practice, there is a very limited research database on such strategies, and these interventions are usually guided by clinical intuition and experience. One issue that is particularly controversial is the use of typical and atypical agents together. This is perhaps most common in people who are on a typical depot medication and an oral atypical. Whilst an anathema to pharmacological purists, and not to be promoted in most cases, some patients do seem to benefit from such combinations and withdrawal of either agent can result in relapse. Many clinicians use other combinations of antipsychotics. In treatment-refractory patients, the combination of clozapine and a 'specific' D2 binding antipsychotic, such as risperidone, sulpiride or amisulpride, has gained some popularity, though there is the potential risk of a greater side-effect burden (Goff et al, 2001).

Another fairly common strategy is to augment with a mood stabilizer, usually either lithium, carbamazepine or sodium valproate, especially in individuals who show an affective component to their illness (Siris, 1993; Barnes et al, 1996; Reutens and Castle, 1997). Such combinations are usually well tolerated and can arguably 'spare' antipsychotics in that the dose required might be lower than if the antipsychotic is used alone (Reutens and Castle, 1997). Lithium can increase the neurotoxicity of antipsychotics, notable clozapine, and thus its use in combination requires caution (Taylor et al, 2001). Carbamazepine can be problematic as it induces the metabolism of a number of hepatic enzymes, thus affecting levels of other drugs; it is also contraindicated with clozapine, due to the propensity to bone marrow suppression.

Evidence that the addition of antidepressants to antipsychotics is useful for enduring negative symptoms is equivocal (Goff et al, 2001). Care needs to be taken with some combinations, e.g. with fluvoxamine and clozapine – the former causes elevations in the serum levels of the latter (Rahman et al, 1998). Also, some tricyclics have been associated with an exacerbation of psychotic symptoms in some individuals. Other augmentation strategies have also been investigated, with mixed results: those targeting negative symptoms are outlined in Chapter 3 and those aiming to enhance cognition in Chapter 4.

Electroconvulsive therapy has also been used in treatment-resistant cases, in combination with antipsychotics, and there is some evidence of additional benefit in terms of antipsychotic effect as well as prevention of relapse (see Rasmussen, 2002). The use of high doses of antipsychotics (above British National Formulary (BNF) guidelines; see Tables 1.1–1.3) is not recommended due to the risk of potentially dangerous side effects (see Morrison, 1996).

Switching antipsychotics

In patients with an established illness and who are well controlled on a typical agent, there is much controversy about whether they should be changed over to atypicals or not. Any change carries with it the possibility of relapse, and patients and their families should be fully informed of this before any such change-over is instituted. Close monitoring of mental state is also required during this phase. Ultimately, the decision about switching depends upon:

- efficacy of current medication, in treating both positive and negative symptoms;
- side effects being experienced; emergent TD is particularly worrisome in patients on typical agents;
- clinical judgement;
- patient preference.

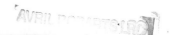

The factors that influence how switches are effected include:

- the current agent and the agent being instituted: e.g. if an agent with powerful sedative effects, such as chlorpromazine, is being replaced with a relatively non-sedative agent, such as risperidone, a supplementary benzodiazepine might be required to cover any rebound insomnia. Similarly, if the established agent has powerful anticholinergic properties (e.g. chlorpromazine, clozapine), judicious short-term use of an anticholinergic agent reduces the risk of cholinergic rebound;
- dose of agent: if the established agent is at high dose, a slower reduction and crossover is preferred, rather than more abrupt discontinuation.

In general, a crossover approach is recommended, rather than discontinuation and then institution of the new agent. This can be effected over days to weeks, depending on the dose and context (e.g. inpatients, who can be closely monitored, can be switched more rapidly). In patients on depots, the usual strategy is to commence the new agent in place of the depot at the time the next depot was due.

The place of depot antipsychotics

Due to problems of adherence amongst patients with schizophrenia and related disorders (see Chapter 8), depot formulations are widely used. These are formulations in an oily base, which should be injected deep into the gluteal muscle, that are effective for 1–4 weeks, depending on the formulation and the individual. The main depot formulations are detailed in Table 1.4. Although a recent meta-analysis (Adams et al, 2001) concluded that there is little to choose between the different depot formulations in terms of efficacy and side effects, some patients do seem to benefit and/or tolerate particular agents better than others, and failure of response and/or intolerable side effects of one depot should not preclude the trial of another.

The problems with depot use include the potential disempowerment of the patient (though some patients prefer depots to oral medication),

References

Adams CE, Fenton MKP, Quraishi S, David AS. (2001) Systematic meta-review of depot antipsychotic drugs for people with schizophrenia. *Br J Psychiatry* **179**: 290–9.

Barnes TRE, McEvedy CJB, Nelson HE (1996). The management of treatment resistant schizophrenia unresponsive to clozapine. *Br J Psychiatry* **169 (Suppl 31)**: 31–40.

Bazire S. (2002) *Psychotropic Drug Directory 2001/02*. (Mark Allen Publishing Ltd: Salisbury).

Bezchlibnyk-Butler KZ, Jeffries JJ (eds). (2001) *Clinical Handbook of Psychotropic Drugs* 11th edn. (Hogrefe & Huber Publishers: Seattle.)

Brown CS, Markowitz JS, Moore TR, Parker NG. (1999) Atypical antipsychotics: Part II adverse effects, drug interactions, and costs. *Ann Pharmacother* **33**: 210–17.

Carson WH, Ali M, Dunbar G, Ingenito G, Saha AR. (2001) A double-blind, placebo-controlled trial of aripiprazole and haloperidol. *Schizophrenia Res* **49**: 221–2.

Davis JM, Metalon L, Watanabe MD, Blake L. (1994). Depot antipsychotic drugs: place in therapy. *Drugs* **47**: 741–73.

Ereshefsky L, Saklad SR, Tran-Johnson T et al. (1990) Kinetics and clinical evaluation of haloperidol decanoate loading dose regimen. *Psychopharmacol Bull* **26**: 108–14.

Goff DC, Freudenreich O, Evins E. (2001) Augmentation strategies in the treatment of schizophrenia. *CNS Spect* **6**: 904–11.

Jibson MD, Tandon R. (1998) New atypical antipsychotic medications. *J Psychiatric Res* **32**: 215–28.

Kane JM. (2000). *Management Issues in Schizophrenia*. (Martin Dunitz: London.)

Kane JM, Eerdekens M, Keith SJ et al. (2002) Efficacy and safety of a novel long-acting risperidone microspheres formulation. *Schizophrenia Res* **53**: 174.

Kane JM, Marder SR. (1993) Psychopharmacologic treatment of schizophrenia. *Schizophrenia Bull* **19**: 287–302.

Kilian JG, Kerr K, Lawrence C, Celermajer DS. (1999) Myocarditis and cardiomyopathy associated with clozapine. *Lancet* **354**: 1841–5.

Kohen D, Bristow M. (1996) Neuroleptic malignant syndrome. *Adv Psychiatr Treat* **2**: 151–7.

Leucht S, Pitschel-Walz G, Engel RR, Kissling W. (2002) Amisulpride, an unusual 'atypical' antipsychotic: a meta-analysis of randomized controlled trials. *Am J Psychiatry* **159**: 180–90.

Lindermeyer J-P. (2000) Treatment refractory schizophrenia. *Psychiatr Quart* **71**: 373–84.

Meltzer HY, Fatemi SH. (1998) Treatment of schizophrenia. In: (Schatzberg AF, Nemeroff CB, eds) *The American Psychiatric Press Textbook of Psychopharmacology*, 2nd Edn. (American Psychiatric Press, Inc: Washington DC) 747–74.

Morrison DP. (1996) Management of treatment refractory schizophrenia. *Br J Psychiatry* **169 (suppl 31)**: 15–20.

Rahman MS, Grace JJ, Pato MT, Priest B. (1998) Setraline in the treatment of clozapine-induced obsessive–compulsive behavior. *Am J Psychiatry* **155**: 1629–30.

Rasmussen KG. (2002) When is ECT indicated in psychiatric disorders? *Curr Psychiatry* **1**: 21–6.

Reutens S, Castle D. (1997) Valproate and neuroleptic medication. *Br J Psychiatry* **170**: 484–5.

Scatton B, Claustre Y, Cudennec A et al. (1997) Amisulpride: from animal pharmacology to therapeutic action. *Int Clin Psychopharmacol* **12** (**suppl. 2**): S29–S36.

Siris SG. (1993) Adjunctive medication in the maintenance treatment of schizophrenia and its conceptual implications. *Br J Psychiatry* **163** (**suppl. 22**): 66–78.

Stahl SM. (1999) Selecting an atypical antipsychotic by combining clinical experience with guidelines from clinical trials. *J Clin Psychiatry* **60** (**suppl. 10**): 31–41.

Taylor D, McConnell H, McConnell H, Kerwin R. (2001). *The Maudsley Prescribing Guidelines*. (Martin Dunitz: London.)

Wagstaff AJ, Bryson HM. (1995). Clozapine: a review of its pharmacological properties and therapeutic use in patients with schizophrenia who are unresponsive to or intolerant of classical antipsychotics. *CNS Drugs* **4**: 37–400.

chapter 2

Psychological approaches to the management of persistent delusions and hallucinations

Til Wykes and David Castle

As more effective treatments for schizophrenia have evolved, emphasis has started to be placed on defining interventions for the individual symptoms rather than on the whole schizophrenia syndrome. The hallmark positive symptoms, i.e. hallucinations and delusions, are a case in point. Although the severity of these symptoms may be controlled by medication, it is not uncommon for them to persist, or at least to reappear in subsequent relapses, despite adequate doses of medication. For some patients the effects of medication on positive symptoms include making them less anxious about the symptoms (this is particularly so for delusions), and allowing them to 'ignore' the symptoms so that they can concentrate on their domestic and social lives. Others describe their 'voices' as getting quieter and less frequent with medication. But for about one third of patients, the positive symptoms continue despite adequate levels of antipsychotic drugs. These symptoms are distressing, and can have dramatic effects on the person's quality of life and on their dependence on psychiatric care.

Symptomatic control by medication also has its costs, expressly at high doses (i.e. side effects), as well as benefits (see Chapter 1). Thus, alternative forms of therapy have been investigated as adjuncts to antipsychotic medication for the control of delusions and hallucinations. Patients and relatives have welcomed these therapies and have put pressure on psychiatric services to provide them as part of a comprehensive service.

The evolution of psychological therapies has been driven by the development of psychological models of the individual symptoms of schizophrenia. Such models have enabled psychologists to establish theories of the mechanisms of the development and maintenance of these symptoms. Together with consideration of the characteristics of these symptoms, such as the levels of conviction for delusions and the physical attributes of the voices, this has led to specific treatment approaches (e.g. Hemsley and Garety, 1986; Frith and Done, 1989; Chadwick and Birchwood, 1994).

Psychological approaches to the reduction of hallucinations

Even though various types of hallucination are experienced by people with schizophrenia, auditory hallucinations are the most prevalent, with around 75% of people with a diagnosis of schizophrenia experiencing them at some stage of their illness (Gelder et al, 1983). The majority of treatment approaches for hallucinations have therefore been aimed at the reduction of this highly prevalent category of abnormal experience. Both cognitive and behavioural approaches have been applied, and more recently there have been attempts to meld the two techniques together. Current techniques are summarized in Table 2.1.

Early interventions were more behavioural in their approach and concentrated on providing competing stimuli that would then divert attention away from the experience of the hallucinations, even including punishment techniques. Even though these interventions can reduce the experience of voices, the effect is usually only a temporary one. In fact, the simple task of keeping a diary of the experiences of hallucinations will, for some people, provide some temporary reduction in the frequency of the hallucinations.

Table 2.1 Psychological interventions for voices

Type of intervention	Therapy	Description
Competing information	Thought stopping	The person has an elastic band around their wrist and is told to snap the elastic band whenever they hear a hallucination, or the person shouts 'Stop it', either overtly or covertly, on occurrence of the voice
	Competing auditory stimuli	Wearing a personal stereo, humming, singing and speaking out loud. Using the muscles involved in vocalization seems to be the most efficacious
	Self-monitoring	Keeping a diary where information is recorded concurrently with the experience. The information includes the thoughts and feelings associated with the experience of the voices
Anxiety reduction	Anxiety management	Carrying out a functional analysis of times of high anxiety then using breathing techniques and relaxation exercises to reduce these experiences. Also, use of systematic desensitization to reduce the impact of specific cues for anxiety
Cognitive	Belief modification	Investigating the events that activate the voice and the consequences. Exploring the content of the voice and providing alternative hypotheses for testing, with exploration of the evidence for the belief
	Focusing	Asking the person to concentrate on the physical attributes of the voices and then gradually encourage identification of the contents of the voice as internally generated
	Coping skills enhancement	Using a case formulation, the person is asked about the antecendents, behaviours and consequences as well as their own coping strategies for dealing with voices

Many psychological approaches to the amelioration of voices also aim to reduce the anxiety associated with them. Slade (1972, 1973) showed that not only did the voices themselves produce anxiety but that anxiety was then often a trigger for the experience of hallucinations. He found that social anxiety in particular was associated with increases in the frequency of hallucinations and that controlling the anxiety in these social situations was associated with a reduction in the experience of voices. He then carried out a series of case studies showing that anxiety management techniques were successful in reducing anxiety and subsequently the experience of hallucinations.

Later interventions developed because of an increased interest in cognition and brain sciences, which produced theories about the relationship between brain functioning and the experience of voices (see Box 2.1). For instance, one theory suggested that hallucinations were the result of poor transfer of information across the corpus callosum, that resulted in a mismatch between the auditory experience in each ear. It was thought that an earplug in the left ear would even up this information transfer and, in fact, those patients who wore an earplug did report significant reductions in voices. However, it was also noticed that some people returned to the clinic with two earplugs, having invested in a further one themselves. Others returned with the earplug in the right ear and also reported reductions in the severity of the hallucinations. It is not clear what was responsible for these reductions but on stopping use of earplugs the voices returned to their usual level (Done et al, 1986).

Although there is no generally accepted psychological model of auditory hallucinations there is an assumption that there is an underlying specific dysfunction in the processing of speech. Some studies using functional neuroimaging suggest that the brain network that is activated when experiencing inner speech is the same one that is activated when people report auditory hallucinations (McGuire et al, 1995). These ideas led to the development of treatments that taught patients to monitor their own speech and encouraged them to reattribute the voices to

Box 2.1 Factors affecting the experience of voices.

Underlying dysfunction in the perception of inner speech (Frith, 1992)
Arousal (induced by social situations or particular stressors)
Beliefs about the voices

themselves (Table 2.1). In a small trial ($n = 6$), Bentall et al (1994) found beneficial effects for half of their patients. However, when Haddock et al (1998) carried out a randomized controlled trial that compared this focusing method with simple distraction, both treatments were found to be equally effective at reducing the frequency of the hallucinations.

As discussed above, anxiety provoking situations appear to increase the frequency of voices. In addition, the patient's level of self-esteem is thought to affect the negative content of the voice. However, there is a third factor that affects the experience of voices – beliefs about the origin and potency of the voices. Birchwood and Chadwick (1997) have shown that the interpretation of the voices – in particular the perceived powerfulness of the voice – affects the severity of the distress experienced. It also seems to be related to behaviour associated with command hallucinations. Changing the beliefs about the powerfulness of the voice has therefore become a further focus for interventions. The therapy of changing beliefs about voices has developed into a more comprehensive treatment intervention called cognitive behaviour therapy (CBT) for hallucinations; this is discussed in more detail below.

Psychological interventions for delusions

For many years it was believed that talking to patients about abnormal beliefs (delusions) was not only unhelpful but could be potentially damaging. Hence, many early therapeutic techniques for delusions entailed trying to distract the person and/or deny them attention whenever they talked about delusional beliefs. These techniques did have the effect of reducing delusional speech, but it has never been clear that there was any accompanying reduction of the ideas themselves rather than patients merely learning to talk about other things, or simply reduce their amount of speech (Liberman et al, 1973).

Some early attempts to try to change patients' beliefs, by discussing them and trying to generate alternative hypotheses about the delusions in collaboration with the patient, proved more successful than challenging the beliefs directly (Watts et al, 1973). This finding led to the development of methods for changing the beliefs themselves. As with psychological interventions for hallucinations, these innovations have been fuelled by an enhanced understanding of the dimensions of delusions, i.e. conviction, preoccupation, interference with everyday life, and distress.

Recently, other factors, e.g. underlying problems with the recognition of the mental states of others (theory of mind), abnormal reasoning biases (particularly jumping to conclusions on little evidence) and the effects of poor self-esteem, have led to more sophisticated therapies. The three current main intervention techniques are given in Box 2.2.

It must be emphasized that the goal of all these techniques is to reduce the negative effects of abnormal beliefs on the lives of people with schizophrenia. Thus, changes in any of the dimensions of the belief will be considered a good outcome. The reason for this is that despite holding abnormal beliefs, i.e. those not considered normal outside of a particular culture, it is possible not to be distressed by them and to be able to continue to manage a reasonable quality of life (Peters et al, 1999).

Box 2.2 Current psychological interventions for delusions.

- **Belief modification**
  Beliefs are ordered into levels of conviction, with the least well-held belief being tackled first, by trying to disentangle the types of evidence used to support the belief and generating alternative explanations.
- **Behavioural experiments**
  These experiments test the veracity of the delusional belief and the supporting evidence.
- **Reattribution**
  This is a more recent therapy, particularly for paranoid ideation, where patients are encouraged to attribute negative events not to people but to situations, with an emphasis on the personal benefits (reduced distress) that these new explanations will bring.

Cognitive behaviour therapy (CBT)

The main developmental roots for CBT have been in understanding and treating depression and anxiety. Two early case studies reported the application of such techniques to schizophrenia (Beck, 1952; Shapiro and Ravenette, 1959), but CBT has only relatively recently been applied more rigorously, through manualized therapies, directly to psychotic symptoms. This development required changes in the presentation of the intervention, although the underlying model of change may be similar to that adopted for mood and anxiety symptoms. The main aims of CBT are to ameliorate distress, disability and emotional disturbance, as well as to reduce the chance of relapse of the acute symptoms (Fowler et al, 1998). CBT employs active and structured therapeutic methods and should be distinguished from psychoeducation, which tends to be simple, didactic and educational. Simple psychoeducation packages have been shown to be ineffective for patients with schizophrenia (Cunningham-Owens et al, 2001) and for their families (Tarrier et al, 1988).

Although there are specific components of CBT that would be accepted by all its proponents, these ingredients may be given in different proportions by different groups of professionals and for different patients. Those elements accepted by most CBT therapists include:

- engagement with the patient;
- problem identification;
- agreeing on a collaborative formulation of the problems to be assessed;
- use of alternative explanations to challenge delusional and dysfunctional thoughts;
- establishing the link between thoughts and emotions;
- encouraging the patient to examine alternative views of events;
- encouraging the patient to examine the link between thoughts and behaviour;
- use of behavioural experiments to reality test;
- setting behavioural goals and targets;
- developing coping strategies to reduce psychotic symptoms;
- development and acquisition of relapse prevention strategies.

Further elements incorporated by some therapists include:

* improvement in self-esteem;
* increasing social support and social networks;
* schema-focused therapy.

What are the outcomes from CBT?

There have now been at least seven randomized control trials of CBT for persistent psychotic symptoms. The majority of participants have been chronic and had medication-resistant symptoms. Many studies, however, have methodological problems such as non-blind rating of symptoms, which is known to inflate measured effectiveness. The studies have adopted different methods for evaluating the efficacy of the therapy, with different rating scales and sometimes idiosyncratic methods of analysis that are difficult to replicate. Despite these reservations, the meta-analyses all suggest that CBT does have an effect on symptom levels that is durable after treatment has been discontinued. The average effect size (the amount of change expected following treatment) is 0.65, which is relatively large. From the three most methodologically rigorous studies (Tarrier et al, 1998, 1999; Kuipers, 1997, 1998; Sensky et al, 2000) there seemed to be overall symptom improvement, although hallucinations appeared more difficult to change than delusions.

A recent study of first- and second-episode patients carried out at the University of Manchester (SoCRATES) evaluated the effect of CBT for patients in the acute phase of their illness. There were small but measurable effects in the first few weeks in the reduction of acute symptoms, particularly hallucinations. However, these short-term effects disappeared as the control conditions caught up with the CBT group. Over an 18-month period following cessation of treatment, improvements in symptom scores were evident, but overall relapse rates were not diminished (Lewis et al, in press).

Most published studies suggest benefit for CBT interventions that last for at least 20 sessions, and are provided by highly trained and supervised therapists. However, there are now trials evaluating the effectiveness of these techniques in normal service settings: there are not yet sufficient data to conclude whether the effects will be similar to those gains made in the earlier studies (Turkington and Kingdon, 2000).

Others investigators have tried to include CBT in a group format to try to increase the number of people with access to the treatment. Wykes et al (1999), in a small exploratory study of CBT for auditory hallucinations, showed that the gains from group treatment were similar to those from individual therapy, although they may not be as durable.

Few studies have evaluated the cost-effectiveness or cost-utility of psychological interventions for the symptoms of schizophrenia, but the available data suggest that the treatments are not very expensive and may even be cost-effective (e.g. Kuipers et al, 1998).

A note about psychological treatments

The success of medication treatments for chronic disorders such as schizophrenia is based on an acute treatment and prevention model, in the same way that diabetes and asthma treatments are evaluated. So, it would be expected that withdrawal of a drug that reduces symptoms would be followed by the return of the symptoms. However, psychological treatment is often evaluated as if it were an antibiotic, with success implying improvements in symptoms and then durability of these changes when the treatment is withdrawn. This leads to the conclusion that if symptoms return following psychological treatment then the treatment has failed. This clearly is not the case – the treatment did affect the symptoms, despite the lack of durability. However, this argument does suggest an alternative regime, i.e. that psychological treatments should also be provided as maintenance therapy given in a 'depot' every few months. These assumptions about treatment mechanisms have seriously hindered the adoption of psychological treatments into health services, because although the maintenance component of the therapy will increase costs, there are likely to be further benefits in terms of quality of life for the patients.

References

Beck AT. (1952) Successful outpatient psychotherapy of a chronic schizophrenic with a delusion based on borrowed guilt. *J Study Interpers Process* **15**: 305–12.

Bentall RP, Haddock G, Slade PD. (1994) Cognitive–behavior therapy for persistent auditory hallucinations – from theory to therapy. *Behav Ther* **25**: 51–66.

Birchwood M, Chadwick P. (1997) The omnipotence of voices: testing the validity of a cognitive model. *Psychol Med* **27**: 1345–53.

Chadwick P, Birchwood M. (1994) The omnipotence of voices: a cognitive approach to auditory hallucinations. *Br J Psychiatry* **164**: 190–201.

Cunningham-Owens DG, Carroll A, Fattah S et al. (2001) A randomised, controlled trial of a brief educational package for schizophrenic out-patients. *Acta Psychiatr Scand* **103**: 362–9.

Done D, Frith C, Owens DC. (1986) Reducing persistent auditory hallucinations through occlusion of monaural input. *Br J Clin Psychol* **25**: 151–2.

Fowler D, Garety P, Kuipers E. (1998) Cognitive therapy for psychosis: formulation, treatment, effects and service implications. *J Ment Health* **7**: 123–33.

Frith CD. (1992) *The Cognitive Neuropsychology of Schizophrenia.* (Lawrence Erlbaum Associates, Inc: Hillsdale, NJ.)

Frith C, Done J. (1989) Positive symptoms of schizophrenia. *Br J Psychiatry* **154**, 569–70.

Gelder M, Gath D, Mayou R. (1983) *The Oxford Textbook of Psychiatry.* (Oxford University Press: Oxford.)

Haddock G, Slade PD, Bentall RP et al. (1998) A comparison of the long-term effectiveness of distraction and focusing in the treatment of auditory hallucination. *Br J Med Psychol* **71**: 339–49.

Hemsley, DR, Garety PA. (1986) The formation of maintenance of delusions: a Bayesian analysis. *Br J Psychiatry* **149**: 51–6.

Kuipers E, Fowler D, Garety P et al. (1998) London–East Anglia randomised controlled trial of cognitive–behavioural therapy for psychosis: III. Follow-up and economic evaluation at 18 months. *Br J Psychiatry* **173**: 61–8.

Kuipers E, Garety P, Fowler D et al. (1997) London–East Anglia randomised controlled trial of cognitive–behavioural therapy for psychosis: 1. Effects of the treatment phase. *Br J Psychiatry,* **171**: 319–27.

Lewis SW, Tarrier N, Haddock G et al. (2002) A randomised controlled trial of cognitive–behaviour therapy in early schizophrenia: acute phase outcomes in the SoCRATES trial. *Br J Psychiatry Suppl* (in press).

Liberman R, Teigen J, Patterson R, Baker V. (1973) Reducing delusional speech in chronic paranoid schizophrenics. *J Appl Behav Anal* **6**: 57–64.

McGuire PK, Silbersweig DA, Wright I et al. (1995) Abnormal monitoring of inner speech – a physiological basis for auditory hallucinations. *Lancet* **346**: 596–600.

Peters ER, Day S, McKenna J, Orbach G. (1999) The incidence of delusional ideation in religious and psychotic populations. *Br J Clin Psychology* **38**: 83–96.

Sensky T, Turkington D, Kingdon D et al. (2000) A randomised controlled trial of cognitive–behavioral therapy for persistent symptoms in schizophrenia resistant to medication. *Arch Gen Psychiatry* **57**: 165–72.

Shapiro MB, Ravenette AT. (1959) A preliminary experiment on paranoid delusions. *J Ment Sci* **105**: 295–312.

Slade PD. (1972) The effects of systematic desensitization on auditory hallucinations. *Behav Res Ther* **10**: 85–91.

Slade PD. (1973) The psychological investigation and treatment of auditory hallucinations: a second case report. *Br J Med Psychology* **46**: 293–6.

Tarrier N, Barrowclough C, Vaughn C et al. (1988) The community management of schizophrenia: a controlled trial of a behavioural intervention with families. *Br J Psychiatry* **153**: 532–42.

Tarrier N, Wittkowski A, Kinney C et al. (1999) The durability of the effects of cognitive behaviour therapy in the treatment of chronic schizophrenia: twelve months follow-up. *Br J Psychiatry* **174**: 500–4.

Tarrier N, Yusupoff L, Kinney C et al. (1998) A randomised controlled trial of intensive cognitive behaviour therapy for patients with chronic schizophrenia. *Br Med J* **317**: 303–7.

Turkington D, Kingdon D. (2000) Cognitive–behavioural techniques for general psychiatrists in the management of patients with psychoses. *Br J Psychiatry* **177**: 101–6.

Watts FN, Powell GE, Austin SV. (1973) The modification of abnormal beliefs. *Br J Med Psychology* **46**, 359–63.

Wykes T, Parr AM, Landau S. (1999) Group treatment for auditory hallucinations – a waiting list controlled study. *Br J Psychiatry* **174**: 180–5.

chapter 3

Management of negative symptoms

David L Copolov and David Castle

As a common source of chronic disability, negative symptoms serve to remind clinicians of the imperfections of psychiatric therapeutics. Negative symptoms are conceptualized as those occurring as a result of a loss of function (Andreasen et al, 1990), including affective flattening, poverty of speech (alogia), diminished drive and loss of pleasure (anhedonia). These symptoms are present to varying degrees in patients with schizophrenia. When present to a significant degree, these symptoms often result in social dislocation and isolation, and greatly reduced activities of daily living.

Just as there is a clear overlap between the positive and negative symptoms of schizophrenia in individual patients, so too do the treatments for these two classes of symptoms overlap – both involve pharmacotherapy, supportive psychotherapy and attention to broader psychosocial issues, such as employment, accommodation and interactions with others. But in dealing with negative symptoms, special emphasis is placed on the consideration of differential diagnoses and on the use of psychosocial rehabilitation strategies.

Negative symptoms are often present from the onset of schizophrenia (Peralta et al, 2000) and usually respond to treatment, but less definitively than positive symptoms (Arndt et al, 1995). It is instructive to subcategorize negative symptoms into phasic negative symptoms that improve in tandem with positive symptoms and enduring negative symptoms. The latter appear to correlate with poor premorbid function, more severe global psychopathology and impaired neuropsychological performance (Tandon et al, 2000). Such enduring negative symptoms are evident even in first episode psychoses (Edwards et al, 1999).

Diagnosis before treatment

There are several important causes of emotional withdrawal, avolition, reduced spontaneity, and reduced affective range in patients with schizophrenia other than the underlying disease processes (Barnes, 1994; Buchanan and Gold, 1996) (Box 3.1).

One such secondary cause is that of **negative symptoms secondary to positive psychotic symptoms.** Hallucinations and delusions may lead to emotional and social withdrawal, both as a response to the often threatening specific content of these psychotic phenomena and to the attempt to reduce external stimuli in the face of being overwhelmed by emotional experiences. During acute psychotic episodes, it may be impossible to distinguish between secondary negative symptoms originating from this cause and primary negative symptoms; such a distinction may be possible only in retrospect.

Negative symptoms due to extrapyramidal side effects (EPSE) of antipsychotic drugs were more common as differential diagnoses with the older generation of antipsychotic drugs (see Chapter 1). But even

Box 3.1 Differential diagnoses of negative symptoms.

Primary negative symptoms
  due to underlying disease processes

Secondary negative symptoms
  secondary to positive psychotic symptoms
  secondary to extrapyramidal side effects (EPSE) of antipsychotic drugs
  secondary to depression
  secondary to catatonia

with atypical drugs in current use, only clozapine and quetiapine carry a very low risk of EPSE (Kapur and Remington, 2001), so this is still an important differential diagnosis to consider. The most obvious feature shared by primary negative symptoms and extrapyramidal syndromes is diminished spontaneous movements (bradykinesia) (Barnes, 1994). Differentiating features therefore focus on the non-bradykinesic set of EPSE symptoms and signs including akathisia, tremor and rigidity. These should be considered when assessing the likelihood that a particular antipsychotic drug might be causing EPSE.

The features of **comorbid depression** that overlap with primary negative symptoms include depressed affect, a reduced capacity for pleasure and decreased engagement with others. Clarification of the differential diagnosis is aided by a detailed consideration of the patient's mood and an enquiry into possible accompanying depressive symptoms, such as recurrent suicidal ideation, persistent insomnia, significant weight loss and intrusive feelings of worthlessness (see Chapter 5). Although there are similarities between flattened and depressed affects, in terms of reduced mobility and range, several studies (Newcomer et al, 1990) have shown that the distinction between these two abnormalities of affect can usually be made reliably, assisted by differentiating features such as tearfulness and observed sadness.

Although **catatonia** is relatively rare in developed countries, it still needs to be kept in mind as a cause of the type of psychomotor inhibition that can be confused with primary negative symptoms (Peralta and Cuesta, 1999). Distinguishing features of catatonia include stupor, bizarre posturing, negativism and waxy flexibility.

Management of negative symptoms

Negative symptoms warrant particular attention from clinicians because they generally fail to give rise to appropriate levels of concern from patients – instead, they tend to engender an attitude of relative indifference (Selten et al, 2000). Thus, clinicians must rely on appropriate and directed history taking, discussion with family members or others who know the patient well, and observation to diagnose and track these symptoms.

The philosophy underlying the diagnosis and treatment of negative symptoms must take into account the fact that, in some circumstances, it may not be possible to distinguish between primary and secondary negative symptoms. Under such circumstances it may be necessary to treat potentially reversible causes of the negative symptoms, such as depression or EPSE, if there is a reasonable level of suspicion that such causes might be relevant to the patient's presentation.

Prevention and management of secondary negative symptoms

The principles underlying the treatment of the positive symptoms of schizophrenia are outlined elsewhere in this book (see Chapters 1 and 2). Treatment of these symptoms will usually result in improvements in negative symptoms, either as a result of *en bloc* improvements in the symptoms of the disorder (with negative symptoms typically improving to a lesser extent than positive symptoms) (Meltzer et al, 2000) or improvements in the negative symptoms that are more directly the consequence of positive ones. One key element of such treatment is the use of antipsychotic drugs. In order to reduce the likelihood of extrapyramidal symptoms arising during the course of treatment with such drugs, the best approach is to choose a novel atypical medication such as quetiapine, olanzapine, ziprasidone or lower dose risperidone, or amisulpride (see Box 3.2). It must be remembered, however, that the risk of EPSE is not uniform across this range of drugs (Collaborative Working Group on Clinical Trial Evaluations, 1998).

If financial considerations preclude the use of newer drugs, then conventional antipsychotic drugs should be used at the lowest effective dose. For haloperidol this dose is likely to be in the range of 3–4 mg daily (McEvoy et al, 1991) or 4–6 mg daily (Nordstrom et al, 1993) – doses which are high enough to achieve the ≥65% dopamine D2 recep-

Box 3.2 Treatment approaches aimed at minimizing
extrapyramidal side effects (EPSE).

Use of newer generation drugs if possible
Lowest effective dose of antipsychotic drugs
Judicious use of anticholinergic medications

tor occupancy levels required for antipsychotic efficacy (Farde et al,
1992, Kapur et al, 1997, 2000).

The trend towards lower antipsychotic dosages is a welcome development but it must be recognized that higher drug doses may need to be
used in order to obtain adequate therapeutic responses. Several groups
have shown that doses in the 200–500 mg chlorpromative equivalents
(CPZ eq) daily range result in greater numbers of responders and that
treatment responsiveness plateaus definitively in the 500–800 mg CPZ eq
daily range (Mossman, 1997). Doses in this latter range are, however,
associated with much higher rates of EPSE; thus, it has been estimated
that to benefit one additional patient in terms of efficacy by treating
with these higher doses will cause significant EPSE in up to four patients
in the first 6 months of maintenance therapy (Mossman, 1997).

Observations such as these have two corollaries. Firstly, there is no
fixed low dose that fits all for each antipsychotic drug and individual
response must be established. Secondly, there are doses below which a
significant percentage of patients do not respond: e.g. in a study of standard versus low-dose fluphenazine decanoate (12.5–50 mg every 2 weeks
versus 1.25–5 mg every 2 weeks), relapse rates over 9 months were eight
times higher (56 versus 7%) in the lower dose group (Kane et al, 1983).
Similarly, studies with risperidone have shown that while there is a rec-
ommendation to start this drug at 2 mg daily (MIMS Australia, 2001),
efficacy is considered to be greatest in the 4–8 mg daily range (Lemmens
et al, 1999); < 2 mg daily, the drug is generally ineffective (Peuskens et al,
1995).

The fact that a substantial number of patients on conventional
antipsychotic drugs (ranging from 20 to 66%; Muscettola et al, 1999)

experience EPSE may therefore be seen as a calculated trade-off of side effects for treatment response. Nevertheless, there is also a high rate of failure to recognize EPSE (Weiden et al, 1986), so vigilance regarding these side effects should always be maintained. If EPSE are detected, either a judicious lowering of the dose to a level sufficient to maintain efficacy, i.e. switching to a drug with less EPSE-causing potential (Weiden et al, 1997), or the addition of anticholinergic drugs such as benzotropine (Holloman and Marder, 1997) should be considered (see Chapter 1). Because of side effects such as dry mouth, blurred vision, constipation, tachycardia and urinary hesitancy, the prophylactic use of anticholinergic agents should be reserved for those being treated with conventional antipsychotic drugs with a history of EPSE, especially those in whom EPSE have led to the discontinuation of antipsychotic medications (Lehman et al, 1998).

The third significant cause of secondary negative symptoms in schizophrenia is depression, the treatment of which is discussed in Chapter 5.

Treatment of primary negative symptoms

There are two elements in treating primary negative symptoms – choosing the most efficacious antipsychotic drug and instigating appropriate psychosocial interventions.

Several reports have claimed efficacy for treating primary negative symptoms with atypical antipsychotic drugs, including olanzapine (Tollefson and Sanger, 1997), risperidone (Möller et al, 1996), amisulpride (Boyer et al, 1995; Paillere-Martinot et al, 1995; Loo et al, 1997) and clozapine (Meltzer, 1992; Breier et al, 1994). Some of these studies have employed path analysis – a statistical technique that factors out the causes of secondary negative symptoms, including EPSE, depression and positive symptoms. Thus, there is suggestive, but far from unequivocal, evidence that newer generation (atypical) antipsychotic drugs have a preferential effect on primary negative symptoms and should therefore be considered first-line treatments when wishing to reduce the likelihood of these symptoms occurring or in treating those in whom these symptoms are prominent. This is compatible with the treatment algorithm outlined in Chapter 1. It should be noted, though, that very few studies have addressed treatment response in patients with the so-called deficit syndrome, in which negative symptoms predominate; further work is required in this area.

Other pharmacological approaches to negative symptoms have included the adjunctive use of glycine (Heresco-Levy et al, 1999), D-cycloserine (Goff et al, 1999; Heresco-Levy et al, 2002), fluvoxamine (Silver and Shmugliakov, 1998), deprenyl (Jungerman et al, 1999) and mirtazapine (Berk et al, 2001). These approaches have yet to be validated.

Psychosocial aspects of managing negative symptoms

A subcomponent meta-analysis and review of 24 psychosocial intervention studies in which negative symptoms had been assessed, demonstrated a greater beneficial effect of such therapies on negative rather than on positive symptoms (Mojtabai et al, 1998). On the basis of chronic patients responding to such treatments better than acute patients, this review also suggested that clinicians adopt a 'phase of illness' orientation to treatment priorities, with priority being given to optimizing medication in the acute phase and to optimizing psychosocial treatments in the chronic phase.

Environmental understimulation is one psychosocial factor that has been shown to exacerbate negative symptoms and is susceptible to intervention. Although research in the long-stay psychiatric institutions of yesteryear provided the data that demonstrated the deleterious role of environmental understimulation (Wing and Brown, 1970), it is just as important to keep track of this factor in the community settings in which patients are now usually treated. The elements comprising environmental understimulation include:

- having little contact with the outside world;
- having little or no engagement in a constructive occupation;
- spending long periods of time doing nothing.

It has been shown that the introduction of measures to address these issues brings substantial benefits in terms of negative symptoms reduction, without a concomitant increase in positive symptoms (Wing and Brown, 1970). In a study of the post-discharge fate of patients who had previously been long-stay (Leff et al, 1994), it has been shown that the provision of enriched social environments is associated with a lessening of negative symptoms, but it may take a number of years for this effect to become evident. Elements that appear to be relevant to improvements in negative symptom status include increase in the number of friends, increased contact with those in the community providing services and goods (such as local shopkeepers), and the provision of less restrictive living environments.

Many of the psychosocial treatments and strategies which are valuable in the management of schizophrenia, such as case management, occupational therapy, assertive community treatment and vocational rehabilitation (see Chapters 4 and 9), attempt to address the negative impact of environmental understimulation on patients. Specific psychosocial interventions that have recently been shown to have some effect on negative symptoms include social skills training (Kopelowicz et al, 1997), group therapy involving multiple families (Dyck et al, 2000), cognitive remediation therapy (Wykes et al, 1999) and cognitive behaviour therapy (Rector and Beck, 2001). The cognitive behaviour therapy of negative symptoms aims to harness motivation, and to promote social and emotional re-engagement by techniques including behavioural self-monitoring, activity scheduling and graded task assignments (Rector and Beck, 2002).

It is important to note the iterative relationship between psychosocial treatments and pharmacotherapy. Antipsychotic medication, such as clozapine, facilitates patient engagement in psychosocial rehabilitation programmes. In turn, these programmes, when used adjunctively with pharmacotherapy, but only after a period of several months, result in additional symptom improvement and a better quality of life (Rosenheck et al, 1998).

Negative symptoms and family members

It is imperative to recognize and help deal with the impact of schizophrenia on family members in the post-deinstitutionalization era, which sees them as the principal caregivers for adults with major psychiatric disorders (see Chapter 10). Family members are often more distressed by the effects of negative symptoms than are the patients themselves (Mueser and Gingerich, 1994). This is especially the case when they have inadequate knowledge about schizophrenia and perceive the symptoms to be under the patient's control (Harrison et al, 1998).

Whether individually or in group settings (Dyck et al, 2000), family members can be helped to cope with negative symptoms in their loved ones (Mueser and Gingerich, 1994). Psychoeducation aimed at clarifying that these symptoms are not the patient's fault is important. **Blunted affect** may lead to a mis-reading of patient's level of interest in activities, so relatives should be advised to ask judiciously about the patient's feelings, rather than assume that impassive facial expressions mean that interest is lacking. One strategy to deal with **poverty of speech** may be to arrange joint activities outside the home. This lessens the pressure on conversation and may provide topics for later discourse. When engaging in discussion, relatives should be encouraging but not place high expectations on what patients can contribute; they should learn to be tolerant of long pauses in conversation and to be active in filling in some of the silences with undemanding contributions. Relatives can help patients with **reduced drive** by regularly scheduling enjoyable recreational activities and making a special effort to include them in family activities.

Conclusions

Negative symptoms are a major contributor to the poor quality of life experienced by patients with schizophrenia (Mueser et al, 1991; Bow-Thomas et al, 1999). While there is a clear need to undertake more research into the pathopsychology of these symptoms in order to improve the limited therapeutic interventions currently available

(Carpenter et al, 1999), there are practical and proven steps that clinicians can take to assist patients deal with secondary and, to a lesser extent, primary negative symptoms.

References

Andreasen NC, Flaum M, Swayze II VW et al. (1990) Positive and negative symptoms in schizophrenia. A critical reappraisal. *Arch Gen Psychiatry* **47**: 615–21.

Arndt S, Andreasen NC, Flaum M et al. (1995) A longitudinal study of symptom dimensions in schizophrenia: prediction and patterns of change. *Am Med Ass* **52**: 352–60.

Barnes TRE. (1994) Issues in the clinical assessment of negative symptoms. *Curr Opin Psychiatry* **7**: 35–8.

Berk M, Ichim C, Brook S. (2001) Efficacy of mirtazapine add on therapy to haloperidol in the treatment of the negative symptoms of schizophrenia: a double-blind randomized placebo-controlled study. *Int J Clin Psychopharmacol* **16**: 87–92.

Bow-Thomas CC, Velligan DI, Miller AL, Olsen J. (1999) Predicting quality of life from symptomatology in schizophrenia at exacerbation and stabilization. *Psychiatry Res* **86**: 131–42.

Boyer P, Lecrubier Y, Puech AJ et al. (1995) Treatment of negative symptoms in schizophrenia with amisulpride. *Br J Psychiatry* **166**: 68–72.

Breier A, Buchanan RW, Kirkpatrick B et al. (1994) Effects of clozapine on positive and negative symptoms in outpatients with schizophrenia. *Am J Psychiatry* **151**: 20–6.

Buchanan RW, Gold JM. (1996) Negative symptoms: diagnosis, treatment and prognosis. *Int Clin Psychopharmacol* **11** **(Suppl 2)**: 3–11.

Carpenter Jr WT, Arango C, Buchanan RW, Kirkpatrick B. (1999) Deficit psychopathology and a paradigm shift in schizophrenia research. *Soc Biol Psychiatry* **46**: 352–60.

Collaborative Working Group on Clinical Trial Evaluations. (1998) Assessment of EPS and tardive dyskinesia in clinical trials. *J Clin Psychiatry* **59** **(Suppl 12)**: 23–7.

Dyck DG, Short RA, Hendryx MS et al. (2000) Management of negative symptoms among patients with schizophrenia attending multiple-family groups. *Psychiatr Serv* **51**: 513–19.

Edwards J, McGorry PD, Waddell FM, Harrigan SM. (1999) Enduring negative symptoms in first-episode psychosis: comparison of six methods using follow-up data. *Schizophrenia Res* **40**: 147–58.

Farde L, Nordstrom AL, Wiesel FA et al. (1992) Positron emission tomographic analysis of central D_1 and D_2 dopamine receptor occupancy in patients treated with classical neuroleptics and clozapine: relation to extrapyramidal side effects. *Arch Gen Psychiatry* **49**: 538–44.

Goff DC, Tsai G, Levitt J et al. (1999) A placebo-controlled trial of D-cycloserine added to conventional neuroleptics in patients with schizophrenia. *Arch Gen Psychiatry* **56**: 21–7.

Harrison C, Dadda M, Smith G. (1998). Family caregivers' criticism of patients with schizophrenia. *Psychiatr Serv* **49**: 918–24.

Heresco-Levy U, Ermilov M, Shimoni J et al. (2002) Placebo-controlled trial of D-cycloserine added to conventional neuroleptics, olanzapine, or risperidone in schizophrenia. *Am J Psychiatry* **159**: 480–2.

Heresco-Levy U, Javitt DC, Ermilov M et al. (1999) Efficacy of high-dose glycine in the treatment of enduring negative symptoms of schizophrenia. *Arch Gen Psychiatry* **56**: 29–36.

Holloman LC, Marder SR. (1997) Management of acute extrapyramidal effects induced by antipsychotic drugs. *Am J Health Syst Pharmacy* **54**: 2461–77.

Jungerman T, Rabinowitz D, Klein E. (1999) Deprenyl augmentation for treating negative symptoms of schizophrenia: a double-blind controlled study. *J Clin Psychopharmacol* **19**: 522–5.

Kane JM, Rifkin A, Woerner M et al. (1983) Low-dose neuroleptic treatment of outpatient schizophrenics. I. Preliminary results for relapse rates. *Arch Gen Psychiatry* **40**: 893–6.

Kapur S, Remington G. (2001) Atypical antipsychotics: new directions and new challenges in the treatment of schizophrenia. *Ann Rev Med* **52**: 503–17.

Kapur S, Zipursky R, Jones C et al. (2000) Relationship between dopamine D(2) occupancy, clinical response, and side effects: a double-blind PET study of first-episode schizophrenia. *Am J Psychiatry* **157**: 514–20.

Kapur S, Zipursky R, Roy P et al. (1997) The relationship between D2 receptor occupancy and plasma levels on low dose oral haloperidol: a PET study. *Psychopharmacology (Berlin)* **131**: 148–52.

Kopelowicz A, Liberman RP, Mintz J, Zarate R. (1997) Comparison of efficacy of social skills training for deficit and nondeficit negative symptoms in schizophrenia. *Am J Psychiatry* **154**: 424–5.

Leff J, Thornicroft G, Coxhead N, Crawford C. (1994) The TAPS Project. 22: a five-year follow-up of long-stay psychiatric patients discharged to the community. *Br J Psychiatry* **165 (Suppl 25)**: 13–17.

Lehman AF, Steinwachs DM, Dixon LB et al. (1998) At issue: translating research into practice: the Schizophrenia Patient Outcomes Research Team (PORT) treatment recommendations. *Schizophrenia Bull* **24**: 1–10.

Lemmens P, Brecher M, Van Baelen B. (1999) A combined analysis of double-blind studies with risperidone vs. placebo and other antipsychotic agents: factors associated with extrapyramidal symptoms. *Acta Psychiatr Scand* **99**: 160–70.

Loo H, Poirier-Littre MF, Theron M et al. (1997) Amisulpride versus placebo in the medium-term treatment of the negative symptoms of schizophrenia. *Br J Psychiatry* **170**: 18–22.

McEvoy JP, Hogarty GE, Steingard S. (1991) Optimal dose of neuroleptic in acute schizophrenia. *Arch Gen Psychiatry* **48**: 739–45.

Meltzer HY (1992) Dimensions of outcome with clozapine. *Br J Psychiatry* **160 (Suppl 17)**: 46–53.

Meltzer H, Kostakaglu E, Lee M. (2000) Response: negative symptoms redux. *Neuropsychopharmacology* **22**: 642–3.

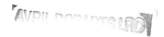

MIMS Australia. (2001) 2001 MIMS Annual. (Vivendi Universal Publishing Co: Sydney for MediMedia Australia Pty Ltd.)

Möller JH, Muller H, Borison RL et al. (1996) A path-analytical approach to differentiate between direct and indirect drug effects on negative symptoms in schizophrenic patients. A re-evaluation of the North American risperidone study. *Eur Arch Psychiatry Clin Neurosci* **245:** 45–9.

Mojtabai R, Nicholson RA, Carpenter BN. (1998) Role of psychosocial treatments in management of schizophrenia: a meta-analytic review of controlled outcome studies. *Schizophrenia Bull* **24:** 569–87.

Mossman D. (1997) A decision analysis approach to neuroleptic dosing: insights from a mathematical model. *J Clin Psychiatry* **58:** 66–72.

Mueser KT, Douglas MS, Bellack AS, Morrison RL. (1991) Assessment of enduring deficit and negative symptom subtypes in schizophrenia. *Schizophrenia Bull* **17:** 565–82.

Mueser KT, Gingerich S. (1994) *Coping with Schizophrenia – A Guide for Families.* (New Harbinger Publications, Inc. Oakland, Ca)

Muscettola G, Barbato G, Pampallona S et al. (1999) Extrapyramidal syndromes in neuroleptic-treated patients: prevalence, risk factors, and association with tardive dyskinesia. *J Clin Psychopharmacol* **19:** 203–8.

Newcomer JW, Faustman WO, Yeh W, Csernansky JG. (1990) Distinguishing depression and negative symptoms in unmedicated patients with schizophrenia. *Psychiatry Res* **31:** 243–50.

Nordstrom AL, Farde I, Wiesel FA et al. (1993) Central D_2-dopamine receptor occupancy in relation to antipsychotic drug effects: a double-blind PET study of schizophrenic patients. *Biol Psychiatry* **33:** 227–35.

Paillere-Martinot ML, Lecrubier Y, Martinot JL, Aubin F. (1995) Improvement of some schizophrenic deficit symptoms with low doses of amisulpride. *Am J Psychiatry* **152:** 130–4.

Peralta V, Cuesta MJ. (1999) Negative, parkinsonian, depressive and catatonic symptoms in schizophrenia: a conflict of paradigms revisited. *Schizophrenia Res* **40:** 245–53.

Peralta V, Cuesta MJ, Martinez-Larrea A, Serrano JF. (2000) Differentiating primary from secondary negative symptoms in schizophrenia: a study of neuroleptic-naïve patients before and after treatment. *Am J Psychiatry* **157:** 1461–6.

Peuskens J and the Risperidone Study Group. (1995) Risperidone in the treatment of patients with chronic schizophrenia: a multi-national, multi-centre, double-blind, parallel-group study versus haloperidol. *Br J Psychiatry* **166:** 712–26.

Rector NA, Beck AT. (2001) Cognitive behavioral therapy for schizophrenia: an empirical review. *J Nerv Ment Dis* **189:** 278–87.

Rector NA, Beck AT. (2002) Cognitive behavioral therapy for schizophrenia: from conceptualization to intervention. *Can J Psychiatry* **47:** 39–48.

Rosenheck R, Tekell J, Peters J et al for the Department of Veterans Affairs Cooperative Study Group on Clozapine in Refractory Schizophrenia. (1998) Does participation in psychosocial treatment augment the benefit of clozapine? *Arch Gen Psychiatry* **55:** 618–25.

Selten J-P, Wiersma D, van den Bosch RJ. (2000) Distress attributed to negative symptoms in schizophrenia. *Schizophrenia Bull* **26:** 737–44.

Silver H, Shmugliakov N. (1998) Augmentation with fluvoxamine but not maprotiline improves negative symptoms in treated schizophrenia: evidence for a specific serotonergic effect from a double-blind study. *J Clin Psychopharmacol* **18:** 208–11.

Tandon R, DeQuardo JR, Taylor SF et al. (2000) Phasic and enduring negative symptoms in schizophrenia: biological markers and relationship to outcome. *Schizophrenia Res* **45:** 191–201.

Tollefson GD, Sanger TM. (1997) Negative symptoms: a path analytic approach to a double-blind, placebo- and haloperidol-controlled clinical trial with olanzapine. *Am J Pscyhiatry* **154:** 466–74.

Weiden PJ, Aquila R, Dalheim L, Standard JM. (1997) Switching antipsychotic medications. *J Clin Psychiatry* **58 (Suppl 10):** 63–72.

Weiden PJ, Shaw E, Mann J. (1986) Causes of neuroleptic non-compliance. *Psychiatr Ann* **16:** 571–8.

Wing JK, Brown GW. (1970) *Institutionalism and Schizophrenia.* (Cambridge University Press: Cambridge.)

Wykes T, Reeder C, Corner J et al. (1999) The effects of neurocognitive remediation on executive processing in patients with schizophrenia. *Schizophrenia Bull* **25:** 291–308.

chapter 4

Cognitive dysfunction in schizophrenia

Til Wykes and David Castle

Cognitive difficulties have been an integral part of the diagnosis of schizophrenia in all diagnostic systems, beginning with Kraepelin and Bleuler more than 100 years ago. However, they differed on the specific mechanism that was at fault; Bleuler emphasized a loosening of the associational threads that tie thoughts together, whilst Kraepelin and others emphasized poor attention and memory difficulties. This chapter describes these difficulties in more detail, with particular reference to the effect they have on quality of life and life choices. Treatment options for cognitive difficulties in schizophrenia are relatively new and have not had their full potential developed; however, details of the most promising of the current therapeutic approaches is provided.

Which cognitive systems are disturbed in schizophrenia?

Impairments are found in a wide range of cognitive systems in people with schizophrenia, but the severity of the impairment differs between systems. For instance, mild impairments are found in overall intelligence quotient (IQ) and for some perceptual tasks; moderate impairments are found for tasks that assess distractibility, delayed recall and working memory; and severe impairments occur in the ability to manipulate information, sometimes called executive functioning (see Table 4.1).

Table 4.1 A profile of cognitive deficits in schizophrenia

Mild	Moderate	Severe
Perceptual skills	Distractibility	Executive functioning
Delayed recognition memory	Memory and working memory	Verbal fluency
Verbal and full scale IQ	Delayed recall	Motor speed

People with schizophrenia are also often very slow in their responses and find it difficult to access a wide vocabulary. There is a distribution of these difficulties within the population of people with schizophrenia with the most severely disabled patients sometimes performing well below average. Of those people who continue to be involved with the psychiatric services, 85% perform below normal on one or more cognitive domains (Harvey and Serper, 1999). In a normal population only 5% have such low levels of functioning, so cognitive deficits can be considered as a core feature of schizophrenia. However, it must be stressed that many people with schizophrenia fall within the normal range of cognitive functioning.

The profile of cognitive deficits found in people with schizophrenia is different to that found in patients with Alzheimer dementia. For example, Alzheimer sufferers have severe impairments in recognition memory but people with schizophrenia are only mildly impaired in these tasks. However, there seems to be only quantitative differences between those with a diagnosis of schizophrenia and those with either bipolar disorder or delusional disorder, with schizophrenia patients being the most disabled.

There has been considerable debate about whether these cognitive difficulties are static or progressive. Studies of birth cohorts and population studies have produced evidence that leaves little doubt about the existence of cognitive difficulties prior to the onset of the disorder. For example, Cannon et al (2002), in a birth cohort from Dunedin, New Zealand, showed that cognitive difficulties at all developmental stages were predictive of the later development of a schizophrenia spectrum disorder when compared to those who later developed other psychiatric disorders or none at all. Lewis et al (2000) also showed, in a cohort of Swedish military, that those who later developed schizophrenia were more likely to have lower IQ than those who did not develop the disorder.

It is also clear that there is a substantial worsening of cognitive performance with the onset of the disorder. Some of the deficits seem to be related to the presence of other symptoms (such as delusions) and remit as symptoms resolve. However, mild difficulties that were evident before the first episode can worsen into a severe cognitive deficit in the months before and during the first episode, and remain relatively stable after remission. For example, memory deficits that may have been mild prior to onset can become severe and hinder all kinds of learning and adaptation to new environmental challenges (Saykin et al, 1994).

Data from cross-sectional studies do not indicate many differences in cognitive functioning between:

- young patients with a short duration of illness, old patients with a short duration of illness and old patients with a long duration of illness (Jeste et al, 1995);
- adolescent and chronic patients (Goldberg and Weinberger, 1988);
- first-episode patients and chronic patients (Albus et al, 1996; Greenwood, 2000).

These data suggest a relative stability of cognitive difficulties over time.

What are the effects of cognitive difficulties on symptoms, rehabilitation and life skills?

Symptoms

It is tempting to assume that cognitive difficulties in schizophrenia are strongly correlated with positive symptoms (hallucinations and delusions), but studies tend to show that cognitive dysfunction accounts for only a small amount of variance in those symptoms. What is clear from high-risk and birth cohort studies is that cognitive difficulties themselves may play a causal role in the propensity for positive symptoms (e.g. Cornblatt et al, 1985). However, it is not yet possible to distinguish within the group of people with schizophrenia the cognitive difficulties that may underpin the severity of specific symptoms. In part, this is due to the lack of subtlety in the measurement of the symptoms themselves. Furthermore, the effect of a cognitive difficulty may only manifest if the cognitive system is stressed so that subtle difficulties, which can be compensated for under normal circumstances, break down. The experiment depicted in Figure 4.1, based on the proposal by Frith (1992) that difficulties in the ability to self-monitor may underlie the experience of hallucinations, demonstrates this. Thus, when asked to distinguish words spoken by themselves or others when they were fed back with distortion of the sound, people with schizophrenia had many more problems in distinguishing their own voice and were biased to say it was someone else's. This difficulty was measurable only when the words were distorted before feeding them back to the patient (Johns et al, 2001).

Rehabilitation

The presence of cognitive difficulties is related to the degree of dependence on psychiatric services, with higher levels of problems being associated with more restrictive forms of care and a lack of independence. The difficulties are also predictive of future care. In a 6-year follow-up study of people who were moved into the community following the closure of a large hospital, cognitive difficulties were a significant predictor of how much care a person would require, such that those with the least impairment were most able to live independently (Wykes and Dunn, 1992). Cognitive difficulties also predict levels of social performance. But perhaps more importantly, cognitive difficulties such as verbal memory problems appear to limit the amount that a person can learn from a traditional rehabilitation programme. Thus, those people with the worst memories achieve the least improvement, particularly in terms of social skills.

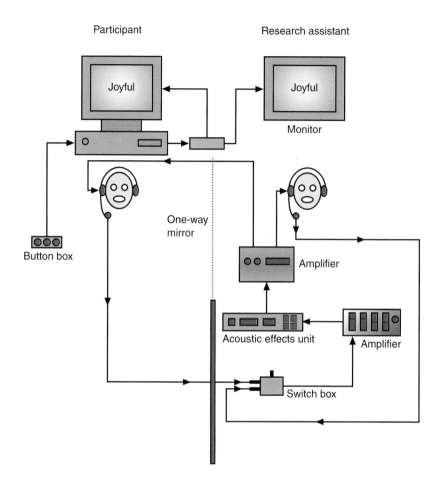

Figure 4.1 *The self-monitoring of voices – the effects of distortion (from Johns et al, 2001). The participant says 'joyful' and then has to decide whether a distorted voice played back to them is theirs or that of another person. Patients who hear voices are biased in thinking that their own voice is an alien one.*

Life skills

Cognitive difficulties not only make a difference to the level of care received but also serve to limit the vocational rehabilitation potential of patients with schizophrenia. Bell et al (2001) have shown that cognition rather than symptoms seems to predict improvements in work quality following a 6-month rehabilitation programme. Gold et al (2001) have also shown that the chance of gaining competitive paid employment following a rehabilitation programme was affected by IQ, memory and speed of processing information. But it must be emphasized that even the most severely cognitively disabled can work if they are provided with the right sort of job and effective support.

Treatment issues

Even though the data suggest that cognitive dysfunctions in schizophrenia tend to be static over time, this does not mean that they are immutable. Indeed, there have been several recent innovative treatment approaches that have now instilled a degree of therapeutic optimism; these are outlined below. What has also been learnt is that some interactions between treatments and cognitive difficulties can make matters worse. For example, when schizophrenia patients with high levels of cognitive difficulties were moved into community placements and had to increase their decision-making, their levels of positive symptoms worsened. In contrast, those without severe cognitive difficulty both improved their social behaviour and showed a reduction in symptoms (Wykes, 1994). It is therefore essential to take into account the current cognitive state of the person when determining treatment plans.

Pharmacological approaches to improving cognition in schizophrenia

Before considering the potential role of medications in ameliorating cognitive deficits in schizophrenia, it is as well to consider how medications might actually worsen cognitive ability. Thus, two of the drugs commonly used for schizophrenia patients, i.e. typical antipsychotics and anticholinergic agents, are known to impair cognition (O'Carroll, 2000). It is important to rationalize the use of such medications and avoid adding to the cognitive impairments that affect so many people with schizophrenia.

In terms of medications that might have a therapeutic effect for cognition in schizophrenia, it is the atypical antipsychotics that have attracted most recent attention. Early reports of an apparent amelioration of cognitive impairment were largely non-randomized within-group switch studies, where patients were assessed prior to and after switching from a typical to an atypical agent. Such a design is flawed in that there is no control for time variables and practice effects, nor for the effect of simply having withdrawn the typical agent. However, recent randomized controlled trials appear to support the notion that atypicals do exert some beneficial effect for cognition, at least relative to typicals (Keefe et al, 1999). One potential confounding effect in the comparison of typicals and atypicals is the lower rate of extrapyramidal side effects (EPSE) with the latter; this would be most marked for tasks requiring manual dexterity. However, it seems that reduced EPSE cannot account for all of the beneficial effect of the atypicals (Green, in press).

What has not been established is the effect of dosage and the time required to establish a positive effect on cognition with atypical antipsychotics. It is also unclear whether particular drugs have effects on particular domains of functioning; e.g. it appears that clozapine improves attention and verbal fluency but has much more equivocal effects on working memory (see Meltzer and McGurk, 1999).

Furthermore, the effect size of improvement in cognition with atypicals is relatively modest and certainly does not compensate for the deficits found in many schizophrenia patients (Green, in press). Put statistically, the extent of improvement in any cognitive domain with the atypical agents is of the order of 0.5 of a standard deviation (SD), whilst the extent of abnormality (see above) is of the order of 2 SD from the normal population mean (see Harvey and Keefe, 2001). Thus, whilst of enormous potential importance, the apparent cognitive benefits of the atypical antipsychotics require a great deal of further careful investigation and do not obviate the need for other strategies such as psychological approaches. These partnership approaches, particularly cognitive remediation plus medication, seem to produce much larger effect sizes that may be clinically significant (Wykes et al, 1999, 2002).

Other pharmacological approaches to enhancing cognition in schizophrenia include the addition of nicotine or psychostimulant drugs. Both of these strategies have shown some promise in enhancing certain cognitive domains, notably attention (see Goff et al, 2001). Further work is required to validate these approaches and establish a role, if any, in clinical practice.

Psychological approaches

Psychological approaches to dealing with cognitive dysfunction in schizophrenia can be divided into three main categories (Box 4.1).

Directly changing cognition

This approach is relatively new and various therapeutic techniques have been adopted to change or improve particular cognitive systems directly. Most have not been very effective but a few have shown improvements that have endured. The large number of non-effective studies has also provided guidance on what not to do. For example, it is now known that only paying people to improve their performance, simply practising a task over and over again, or merely simplifying the task are all ineffective (Wykes and van der Gaag, 2001).

The most robustly effective approach is called cognitive remediation therapy (CRT) (Wykes and Van der Gaag, 2001). This therapy does not simply teach tasks, but it concentrates on providing strategies for dealing with problems in general. What seems to be essential is to

---

Box 4.1 Main psychological approaches.

- Direct approaches where the cognitive difficulty is the target of the rehabilitation;
- Changing the rehabilitation programme so that it plays to the strengths rather than weaknesses of the patient;
- Changing the environment so that it compensates for the cognitive deficits.

provide tasks where patients learn to achieve goals through their own efforts; this is termed self-efficacy. This requires the provision of tasks that are just inside the patient's level of competence, so that they have to make some learning effort but do succeed. Reducing the number of errors made by the patient (errorless learning) is also essential, as people with schizophrenia find it hard to distinguish in their memory between responses that produced errors and responses that were correct. Thus, if they make many errors they will not be able to carry out the task correctly at a later date. The studies that have been carried out so far have used paper-and-pencil tasks or computer games to teach information processing skills and are usually supervised by clinical psychologists, but Table 4.2 shows the sort of approaches that could be provided within any psychosocial treatment programme.

Changing rehabilitation programmes to fit strengths

It seems obvious that cognitive difficulties need to be taken into account in providing any psychosocial rehabilitation programme. This means obtaining a profile of the cognitive difficulties of a person and then using this to guide the design of an individualized programme. For example, poor verbal memory is known to limit learning in a social skills training programme. The most sensible response is to change the programme itself so that it does not rely too heavily on verbal memory. This sort of approach has been adopted in the learning disability literature but has not been investigated extensively in programmes for people with schizophrenia.

Changing the environment

This is the last resort for the treatment of cognitive difficulties, and is similar to the approaches made for people with dementia or a head injury. Here, the environment is changed so that there is less demand on the dysfunctional cognitive systems. One randomized trial in Texas showed that by providing this sort of support patients with cognitive difficulties improved their overall functioning (Velligan et al, 2000). The key worker/case manager visits the person at least twice a week and provides a series of cues for carrying out particular tasks, such as alarms to

Table 4.2 Cognitive enhancement strategies for people with schizophrenia

Life skill	Cognitive skills required	Useful strategies to aid relevant cognitive skills	Useful tasks to target relevant skills
Shopping for groceries	Planning Memory Sequencing	Write a shopping list or repeat to yourself what you need to buy Break the shopping list into categories Order your list according to the layout of the shop(s)	Devising a plan for how to implement a problem-solving task Reordering numbers from a disorganized list Memorizing a set of words
Reading a train timetable	Attention to detail Shifting attention Self-monitoring	Check details frequently Trace along lines with fingers to avoid visual neglect Use verbal mediation to remind yourself what you are looking for	Searching through a grid of letters for changing target letters Line bisection tasks (estimating the midpoint of a line)
Remembering the route to the shop	Spatial memory	Visualize the route Generate a verbal description Use verbal repetition Associate landmarks with familiar objects Make a list of landmarks Draw yourself a map	Memorizing sequences of squares on a grid Memorizing designs Generating verbal descriptions for designs or sequenced patterns

Table 4.2 continued

Life skill	Cognitive skills required	Useful strategies to aid relevant cognitive skills	Useful tasks to target relevant skills
Planning your next move in a game of draughts	Spatial memory Planning Sequencing	Visualize the moves Find visual patterns to describe the moves Generate a verbal description for the moves Use verbal repetition	Visual transformation tasks (e.g. draw what this shape would look like if it was rotated by half a turn) Memorizing geometric patterns Memorizing sequences of moves on a grid
Holding a conversation in a noisy room	Auditory verbal memory Comprehension Selective attention Self-monitoring	Minimize distractions Ask the other person to repeat what they said Don't rush what you are saying	Generating verbal descriptions for pictures Listening to instructions and then carrying them out Answering questions about a spoken passage Counting target items whilst tapping a sequence with your hand

Table 4.2 *continued*

Life skill	Cognitive skills required	Useful strategies to aid relevant cognitive skills	Useful tasks to target relevant skills
Reading a magazine article	Verbal comprehension Verbal memory Attention to detail	Use chunking Use repetition Follow each line with your finger to ensure nothing is missed out and reading speed is not too fast	Comprehension tasks – learning a written passage and answering questions about it Searching for target letters or numbers in a grid
Baking a cake using a recipe	Sustained attention Shifting attention Sequencing Planning Memory Self-monitoring	Take one step at a time Organize your equipment Use written records Use verbal repetition Devise a plan before you begin Create subgoals Check steps as you proceed	Attentional shifting tasks (e.g. copying a design onto another sheet of paper) Sequencing tasks – describe the steps needed to carry out problem-solving tasks

remind them when to go out to the day centre. They also organize their activities minutely, e.g. placing all the clothes required for a single day into boxes and labelling them with the days of the week; the person then puts on all the clothes for that particular day, no more and no less (Velligan et al, 2000). This form of therapy, known as cognitive adaptational training, could be seen as rather intrusive and may not be acceptable to some services and patients.

Conclusions

Cognitive impairments are common in schizophrenia and mediate much of the disability experienced by people with the condition. Atypical antipsychotics may be associated with some degree of improvement in cognition and certain novel psychological therapies show promise in terms of ameliorating cognitive deficits.

References

Albus M, Hubmann W, Ehrenberg C et al. (1996) Neuropsychological impairment in first-episode and chronic schizophrenic patients. *Eur Arch Psychiatry Clin Neurosci* **246**: 249–55.

Bell M, Bryson G, Tamasine G et al. (2001) Neurocognitive enhancement therapy with work therapy: effects on neuropsychological test performance. *Arch Gen Psychiatry* **58**: 763–8.

Cannon M, Caspi A, Moffitt TE et al. (2002) Evidence for early-childhood, pandevelopmental impairment specific to schizophreniform disorder: results from a longitudinal birth cohort. *Arch Gen Psychiatry* **59**: 449–57.

Cornblatt BA, Lenzenweger MF, Dworkin RH, Erlenmeyer-Kimling L. (1985) Positive and negative schizophrenic symptoms, attention, and information processing. *Schizophrenia Bull* **11**: 397–408.

Frith C. (1992) *The Cognitive Neuropsychology of Schizophrenia.* (Lawrence Erlbaum Associates: Hove, East Sussex.)

Goff DC, Freudenreich O, Evins AE. (2001) Augmentation strategies in the treatment of schizophrenia. *CNS Spect,* **6**: 904–11.

Gold J, Iannone V, McMahon R, Buchanon R. (2001) Cognitive correlates of competitive employment among patients with schizophrenia. *Schizophrenia Res* **49**: 134.

Goldberg TE, Weinberger DR. (1988) Probing prefrontal function in schizophrenia with neuropsychological paradigms. *Schizophrenia Bull* **14**: 179–83.

Green MF. (2002) Recent studies on the neurocognitive effects of second generation antipsychotic medications. *Curr Opin Psychiatry* **15**: 25–9.

Greenwood K. (2000) *The nature and stability of executive impairments in schizophrenia.* PhD Thesis, University of London.

Harvey PD, Keefe RSE. (2001) Studies of cognitive change in patients with schizophrenia following novel antipsychotic treatment. *Am J Psychiatry* **158**: 176–84.

Harvey P, Serper M. (1999) The nature and management of cognitive dysfunction in patients with schizophrenia. *Direct Psychiatry* **19**: 21–35.

Jeste DV, Harris MJ, Krull A et al. (1995) Clinical and neuropsychological characteristics of patients with late-onset schizophrenia. *Am J Psychiatry* **152**: 722–30.

Johns LC, Rossell S, Frith C et al. (2001) Verbal self-monitoring and auditory verbal hallucinations in patients with schizophrenia. *Psychol Med* **31**: 705–15.

Keefe RSE, Silva SG, Perkins DO, Lieberman JA. (1999) The effects of atypical antipsychotic drugs on neurocognitive impairment in schizophrenia: a review and meta-analysis. *Schizophrenia Bull* **25**: 201–22.

Lewis G, David AS, Malmberg A, Allebeck P. (2000) Non-psychotic psychiatric disorder and subsequent risk of schizophrenia: cohort study. *Br J Psychiatry* **177**: 416–20.

Meltzer HY, McGurk SR. (1999) The effects of clozapine, risperidone, and olanzapine on cognitive function in schizophrenia. *Schizophrenia Bull* **25**: 233–55.

O'Carroll R. (2000) Cognitive impairment in schizophrenia. *Adv Psychiatr Treat* **6**: 161–8.

Saykin AJ, Shtasel DL, Gur RE et al. (1994) Neuropsychological deficits in neuroleptic naive patients with first-episode schizophrenia. *Arch Gen Psychiatry* **51**: 124–31.

Velligan DI, Bow-Thomas CC, Huntzinger CD et al. (2000) A randomized controlled trial of the use of compensatory strategies in schizophrenic outpatients: cognitive adaptation training. *Am J Psychiatry* **157**: 1317–23.

Wykes T. (1994) Predicting symptomatic and behavioural outcomes of community care. *Br J Psychiatry* **165**: 486–92.

Wykes T, Dunn G. (1992) Cognitive deficit and the prediction of rehabilitation success in a chronic psychiatric group. *Psychol Med* **22**: 389–98.

Wykes T, Reeder C, Corner J et al. (1999) The effects of neurocognitive remediation on executive processing in patients with schizophrenia. *Schizophrenia Bull* **25**: 291–308.

Wykes T, Reeder C, Williams C et al. (2002) Are the effects of cognitive remediation therapy (CRT) durable? Results from an exploratory trial. *Schizophrenia Res* (in press).

Wykes T, Van Der Gaag M. (2001) Is it time to develop a new cognitive therapy for psychosis – Cognitive Remediation Therapy (CRT)? *Clin Psychol Rev* **21**: 1227–56.

chapter 5

Depression and anxiety in schizophrenia

David Castle and Til Wykes

The extent of psychiatric comorbidity in schizophrenia is often not appreciated, in part this is because of a heritage of an essentially hierarchical approach to psychiatric diagnosis, where schizophrenia trumps depression and anxiety. However, the recognition of depressive and anxiety symptoms in people with schizophrenia is important, as these symptoms are common, tend to worsen the longitudinal course of illness, and can result in secondary morbidity and suicide. This chapter provides a brief overview of depression and selected anxiety disorders (social anxiety and obsessive–compulsive disorder) in schizophrenia.

Depression and schizophrenia

The relationship between schizophrenia on the one hand and affective disorders on the other has dominated the nosological debate for well over a century, ever since Kraepelin's (1893) original dichotomization of dementia praecox from manic depression. Bleuler (1911), who coined the term schizophrenia, included affective symptoms (anhedonia) in his definition of the disorder. But it was Kasanin (1933), in describing patients with what he called schizoaffective disorder, who shifted the debate to a consideration of patients with an admixture of both schizophrenic and affective symptoms; the place of such disorders in the nosology is still debated (see Levinson et al, 1999). Here, schizoaffective disorders are not considered as such, nor are manic psychoses addressed; instead concentration is on depression in people with schizophrenia. For reviews of the treatment of schizoaffective disorder see Azorin (1995) and Levinson et al (1999).

It is not uncommon for people with schizophrenia to manifest depressive symptoms. Indeed, the National Comorbidity Survey in the USA reported that 59% of people with schizophrenia also had a lifetime diagnosis of depression. In clinical samples of schizophrenia patients, rates of depression of anything from 7 to 65% have been reported, dependent upon the clinical sample and the definition of depression; Siris (1991), who reviewed these studies, suggested a modal figure of 25%.

The extent of this comorbidity is, in many ways, unsurprising, as many people with schizophrenia suffer from secondary social dysfunction, including the break-up of families and relationships, loss of study/work, and poverty (see Box 5.1). Such factors are associated with depression in the general population. Furthermore, schizophrenia is a severe and long-term illness which carries with it considerable stigma, thus it is difficult for the patient to adjust to.

Effect of depression on the longitudinal course of schizophrenia

Some early studies suggested that depression in schizophrenia might be a predictor of favourable outcome. However, such studies were almost certainly confounded by the inclusion of people with schizoaffective

Box 5.1 Factors that might mediate depression in schizophrenia.

Social factors (unemployment, lack of social network, etc.)
Psychosocial stressors (e.g. loss of role, family stress)
Adjustment to diagnosis
Alcohol and illicit substance use
Non-compliance with antipsychotic medication
Direct dysphoric effect of antipsychotic medication
Extrapyramidal side effects of antipsychotic medication

disorders and it is now generally accepted that depression worsens the long-term course of schizophrenia (Siris, 1995).

What is undoubtedly the case is that rates of completed suicide are far higher in schizophrenia patients than the general population (around 10% of people with schizophrenia die by suicide). In a single year, 3800 schizophrenia sufferers in the USA committed suicide (Jones et al, 1994). There is a strong correlation between depressive symptoms, notably hopelessness, and suicide in schizophrenia (Jones et al, 1994); thus, it is imperative that clinicians recognize and treat depression in those with this condition.

Recognising depression in schizophrenia

One of the impediments to the recognition of depression in people with schizophrenia is the diagnostic hierarchy alluded to above. Thus, clinicians tend to concentrate on eliciting and monitoring psychotic symptoms, rather than depression. The problem is made worse by the fact that both psychotic symptoms and side effects of antipsychotic medication can manifest very much like depression, and the distinction can be difficult to make (see Box 5.2).

For example, depressive lack of motivation and interest can be confused with the apathetic social withdrawal of schizophrenia, or it might be considered a sign of demoralization (Frank, 1973). Andreasen (1998) suggests that the eliciting of vegetative symptoms, such as anorexia or insomnia, or expressions of low self-esteem and guilt should sway the diagnosis towards one of depression (see also Chapter 3).

Box 5.2 Psychotic symptoms and antipsychotic side effects presenting as depression.

Positive psychotic symptoms
Negative symptoms
Akinesia
Akathisia

Another factor to consider is that antipsychotic agents can produce side effects that can mimic depression. **Akinesia** can be missed clinically, as it does not always occur in the setting of obvious parkinsonism (Van Putten and May, 1978). **Akathisia** is also associated with mood symptoms, notably dysphoria, and has been linked with suicide (Drake and Ehrlich, 1985). Such side effects are important to recognize and treat, as outlined below.

Do antipsychotics cause depression?

There is considerable debate about whether antipsychotics actually cause depression. Siris (1991), in weighing the evidence, points to three sets of findings that suggest this is not a major factor.

- Depressive symptoms tend to improve as psychotic symptoms improve.
- Similar rates of depression have been reported in schizophrenia patients on and off antipsychotics.
- Studies have failed to show any consistent correlation between depressive symptoms and antipsychotic dose or plasma level.

However, other authors refute this conclusion and have suggested a role for antipsychotic-mediated effects on dopamine-mediated reward systems in the brain as aetiologically important (Harrow et al, 1994).

Any dysphoric effect of antipsychotics is not likely to be prominent with the newer atypical agents (see Chapter 1). Indeed, risperidone, olanzapine and ziprasidone have all been shown to have antidepressant effects in schizophrenia patients (see Siris, 2000). It is supposed that this is dictated by the serotonergic actions of these drugs, although a number of other parameters should also be considered (see Box 5.3). In an important study that controlled for the effects of lower extrapyramidal side effects (EPSE) with olanzapine compared with haloperidol, Tollefson et al (1998) employed path analysis to show a direct antidepressant effect of olanzapine.

Treating depression in schizophrenia

Box 5.4 presents some factors that should be excluded in schizophrenia

Box 5.3 Ways in which atypical antipsychotics may produce antidepressant effects.*

Tend not to produce extrapyramidal side effects at therapeutic doses
Tend not to produce neuroleptic-induced deficit symptoms
More efficacy against negative symptoms (notably clozapine)
Reduce illicit substance use
Enhance compliance with medication
Enable more effective psychosocial rehabilitation, including work
Direct antidepressant effect

* Based on Siris (2000).

patients presenting with depression. Some of these might require a therapeutic trial, e.g. an anticholinergic challenge if akinesia is suspected, or propranolol or a benzodiazepine in patients with akathisia. It is also important to recognize that there is little evidence for the efficacy of antidepressant medication for dysphoria in patients who have prominent positive symptoms of psychosis and the priority should be the optimal control of psychotic symptoms (Siris, 1991).

Box 5.4 Factors to exclude in schizophrenia patients presenting with depression.*

Organic disorders (medical)
Alcohol abuse
Illicit substance use
'Pre-psychotic' prodromal phase of psychotic episode
Negative symptoms (e.g. anergia, apathetic social withdrawal)
Schizoaffective depression
Antipsychotic side effects (notably akinesia and akathisia)
Demoralization (diminished sense of subjective control over the illness)

*Based on Siris (1991, 2000).

Psychological strategies

The treatment of depression in schizophrenia requires a multifaceted biopsychosocial approach. Life events resulting from an acute episode, the stigma attached to the illness as well as the loss of social roles are known to be associated with depression in schizophrenia (Birchwood and Iqbal, 1998). Psychological factors associated with psychotic symptoms are also likely to predict depression. For instance, the degree of malevolence of the content of an auditory hallucination and the powerfulness of the voice are predictive of depression.

The overall strategy should therefore be to encourage a blame-free acceptance of the illness and a mastery of illness (see Birchwood and Iqbal, 1998). A cognitive approach to symptoms and the appraisal of the self would therefore have an impact on depression. There is, however, little empirical evidence to support any specific psychological therapy. Thus, interventions should be tailored to the particular needs of the individual within the overall model; e.g. grief work should be provided for those experiencing loss, and rehabilitation and resocialization programmes for those manifesting demoralization.

Pharmacological strategies

In terms of medication, it appears clear from the discussion above that atypical antipsychotics will come to play an important role in the treatment of depression in schizophrenia. Siris (2000) reviewed 13 prospective randomized controlled trials of atypical antipsychotics in schizophrenia, and found that 12 of these reported antidepressant efficacy. Thus, atypical antipsychotics seem a prudent choice in the setting of schizophrenia complicated by depression. An effect on suicidality would also be expected, which has been confirmed for clozapine (Meltzer and Okayli, 1995).

The evidence regarding the addition of antidepressants to antipsychotics is rather mixed and some studies have reported a worsening of psychotic symptoms with this combination. In reviewing this literature, Levinson et al (1999) found 'substantial evidence' for the efficacy of the addition of an antidepressant in schizophrenia patients who develop a full major depressive syndrome after resolution of psychosis.

The evidence regarding depressive symptoms not meeting syndromic 'caseness' is equivocal, and in this setting strategies such as optimization of antipsychotic treatment and psychosocial interventions should be considered prior to resorting to antidepressant medication. If antidepressants are added, their effect on mood requires close monitoring of overall symptomatology; worsening of psychotic symptoms might require their withdrawal.

Dufresne (1995) provided a useful overview of the potential problems arising from the addition of antidepressants to antipsychotic drugs in general. These problems include pharmacodynamic and pharmacokinetic effects that can exacerbate side effects, such as the combination of two agents with anticholinergic or cardiotoxic effects. Common sense should prevail in choosing which combination of drugs to use and side effects should be monitored carefully, with drug levels being checked for combinations that affect each other's metabolism. In clinical practice, selective serotonin reuptake inhibitors (SSRI) are often added to atypical antipsychotics in patients with persistent depression; a combination which is usually well tolerated. The addition of lithium to an antipsychotic and the place of electroconvulsive therapy in depression in schizophrenia have not been adequately studied, although may be indicated in particular patients.

Anxiety disorders in schizophrenia

It is often assumed that symptoms of anxiety in people with schizophrenia are secondary to positive psychotic symptoms (i.e. delusions and hallucinations). However, a number of studies have now confirmed substantial anxiety comorbidity in schizophrenia, not merely consequent upon positive symptoms. For example, Cassano et al (1998) found, in their sample of 31 patients with schizophrenia spectrum disorders, that 58% were comorbid for another Diagnostic and Statistical Manual (DSM)-IIIR psychiatric disorder; 19% had a lifetime diagnosis of panic disorder, 29% obsessive–compulsive disorder (OCD) and 16% social phobia. In another study of patients with schizophrenia ($n = 60$),

Casoff and Hafner (1998) found 12% were comorbid for generalized anxiety disorder, 13% for OCD and 17% for social phobia. Similarly, Goodwin et al (2001) reported a rate of 15% for panic attacks in their sample of 120 people with psychotic disorders.

A fairly consistent finding is that anxiety comorbidity in schizophrenia is associated with a relatively worse illness outcome. For example, Goodwin et al (2001) found that psychosis patients with panic comorbidity fared worse on outcomes such as psychiatric symptomatology, rehabilitation outcome and quality of life than their counterparts without panic. It is also the case that the anxiety comorbidity often goes unrecognized and hence is not directly treated (Casoff and Hafner, 1998). It is important that all the experiences of schizophrenia patients are not dismissed as being part of their psychotic illness, as the mere acknowledgement of anxiety symptoms as non-psychotic can be both reassuring and empowering for the patient.

Social phobia

Some degree of impairment of social functioning is not unusual in schizophrenia. This might be secondary to positive symptoms, to negative symptoms or to the disruption of social maturation and adeptness that the early onset of a severe psychiatric disorder can bring. These problems are compounded by stigmatization and negative attitudes in the general population regarding schizophrenia.

It is often assumed that social dysfunction in schizophrenia is part and parcel of the illness process, and that little can be done to ameliorate it: this is not the case. Indeed, social skills training has a track record in rehabilitation of schizophrenia, although it is not effective for all patients and when gains do accrue they often cannot be applied to new situations (Wallace et al, 1980). Furthermore, it is often the case that social phobia as such is not considered as a dependent variable in investigations of social skills training (see Penn et al, 1994). However, some studies are beginning to investigate social anxiety in schizophrenia patients directly. One successful controlled trial (Halperin et al, 2000) employed a group-based cognitive–behavioural therapy (CBT) intervention, an outline of which is shown in Box 5.5. This study reported gains in terms of social anxiety, mood, and overall quality and enjoyment of life. Important further steps will be to determine precisely which elements of this sort of intervention are effective, and then to integrate those elements into social skills training packages.

Obsessive/compulsive disorder

The co-occurrence of OCD and schizophrenia has been recognized for decades but has been the principal subject of few investigations (see Dowling et al, 1995). Indeed, Fabisch et al (2001) could find only nine studies since 1926 that directly investigated the prevalence of obsessive–compulsive (OC) symptoms in schizophrenia. Reported rates varied widely (anything from 1 to 54%), depending on sample selection and the diagnostic criteria employed. All studies found that OC symptoms tended to antedate psychotic ones. In one of the most methodologically

---

Box 5.5 Outline of group-based programme for social phobia in schizophrenia.*

Session 1. Overview of anxiety – social anxiety in particular; sharing of experiences/concerns by group members; setting objectives and first homework tasks (e.g. social exposure tasks, with monitoring and challenging of unhelpful automatic thoughts)

Session 2. Review of previous week and of homework; introduction to cognitive restructuring, including challenging negative automatic thoughts

Session 3. Exposure exercise, with role play; review of cognitive restructuring

Session 4. Educational video on social phobia; further homework assignments

Sessions 5–7. Homework reviews, cognitive restructuring with increasing onus on participants to take initiative

Session 8. Social outing; closure and future individual planning

---

*Based on Halperin et al (2000).

sound of these studies, Eisen et al (1997) found that six (7.7%) of 77 patients with schizophrenia or schizoaffective disorder also met DSM-IIIR criteria for OCD; this rate is 2–3 times that reported in general population samples.

The reasons for the coaggregation of OC symptoms and psychotic symptoms have not been established. Stengel (1945) believed that the occurrence of such features were to some degree protective against 'personality disintegration' in schizophrenia, but more recent studies suggest that schizophrenia patients with OC symptoms actually have a worse longitudinal outcome than their counterparts without such symptoms. For example, in the Chestnut Lodge 16-year follow-up of chronic schizophrenia patients, those with OC symptoms had a particularly poor outcome in terms of psychopathology, social and occupational functioning, and global outcome (Fenton and McGlashan, 1986). Fenton and McGlashan (1986) offer the following possible explanatory hypotheses:

* There is a specific subtype of schizophrenia with OC symptoms, which has a pernicious course.
* Patients exhibiting schizophrenia and OC symptoms have two comorbid disorders, which additively contribute to a poor prognosis.
* Early onset of OCD impairs the individual's social development and thus contributes to social disability when schizophrenia manifests.

Treatment of OCD in schizophrenia
The treatment of OC symptoms in schizophrenia has not been adequately studied. Clinicians tend to rely on the compelling evidence of the efficacy of serotonergic antidepressants (clompiramine, SSRI) in uncomplicated OCD (see Hood et al, 2001) and employ these in comorbid cases in addition to antipsychotic therapy (Goff et al, 1990; Zohar et al, 1993). The use of behavioural therapy for OC symptoms in schizophrenia requires scientific study, but anecdotal evidence is that it can be employed effectively in such patients and may obviate the need for polypharmacy.

A curious issue which has arisen with the advent of the atypical antipsychotics, notably clozapine (see Chapter 1) is the tendency of such agents to exacerbate or produce *de novo* OC symptoms (see Hood et al, 2001). The putative mechanism implicates the serotonin (5HT) actions of these agents, although this has not been rigorously tested. Irrespective, it appears that the treatments outlined above (i.e. serotonergic antidepressants and behavioural therapy) can be effectively employed in this clinical scenario and discontinuation of the atypical antipsychotic is not usually necessary (e.g. Dowling et al, 1995).

Conclusions

Depression and anxiety are common in patients with schizophrenia, and are often associated with a worsening of the long-term illness outcome. It is important that such symptoms are recognized and adequately treated.

References

Andreasen NC. (1998) Mood disorders and schizophrenia. *J Clin Psychiatry* **16:** 7–8.

Azorin J-M. (1995) Long-term treatment of mood disorders in schizophrenia. *Acta Psychiatr Scand* **91 (Suppl 388):** 20–3.

Birchwood M, Iqbal I. (1998) Depression and suicidal thinking in psychosis. In: (Wykes T, Tarrier N, Lewis S, eds) *Innovation and Outcome in Psychological Treatment of Schizophrenia* (Wiley: Chichester) 81–118.

Bleuler E. (1911) *Dementia. Praecox or the group of Schizophrenia.* Translated by J Zinkin. (International Universities Press: New York, 1950).

Casoff SJ, Hafner J. (1998) The prevalence of comorbid anxiety in schizophrenia, schizoaffective disorder and bipolar disorder. *Aust NZ J Psychiatry* **32:** 67–72.

Cassano GB, Pini S, Saettoni M et al. (1998) Occurrence and clinical correlates of psychiatric comorbidity in patients with psychotic disorders. *J Clin Psychiatry* **59:** 60–8.

Dowling FG, Pato MT, Pato CN. (1995) Comorbidity of obsessive–compulsive and psychotic symptoms: a review. *Harvard Rev Psychiatry* **3:** 75–83.

Drake RE, Ehrlich J. (1985) Suicide attempts associated with akathisia. *Am J Psychiatry* **142:** 499–501.

Dufresne RL. (1995) Issues in pharmacotherapy: focus on depression in schizophrenia. *Psychopharmacol Bull,* **31:** 789–96.

Eisen JL, Beer DA, Pato MT et al. (1997) Obsessive compulsive disorder in patients with schizophrenia or schizoaffective disorder. *Am J Psychiatry* **154:** 271–3.

Fabisch K, Fabisch H, Langs G et al. (2001) Incidence of obsessive–compulsive phenomena in the course of acute schizophrenia and schizoaffective disorder. *Eur Psychiatry* **16**: 336–41.

Fenton WS, McGlashan TH. (1986) The prognostic significance of obsessive–compulsive symptoms in schizophrenia. *Am J Psychiatry* **143**: 437–41.

Frank JD. (1973) *Persuasion and healing.* (John Hopkins University Press: Baltimore).

Goff DC, Brotman AW, Waiters M, McCormick S. (1990) Trial of fluoxetine added to neuroleptics for treatment resistant schizophrenia patients. *Am J Psychiatry* **147**: 492–4.

Goodwin R, Stayner DA, Chinman MJ, Davidson L. (2001) Impact of panic attacks on rehabilitation and quality of life among persons with severe psychotic disorders. *Psychiatr Serv* **52**: 920–4.

Halperin S, Nathan P, Drummond P, Castle D. (2000) A cognitive–behavioural group-based treatment for social anxiety in schizophrenia. *Aust NZ J Psychiatry* **34**: 809–13.

Harrow M, Yonan C, Sands JR, Marengo J. (1994) Depression in schizophrenia: are neuroleptics, akinesia, or anhedonia involved? *Schizophrenia Bull* **20**: 327–38.

Hood S, Alderton D, Castle DJ. (2001) Obsessive–compulsive disorder: treatment and treatment resistance. *Australas Psychiatry* **9**: 118–27.

Jones JS, Stein DJ, Stanley B et al. (1994) Negative and depressive symptoms in suicidal schizophrenics. *Acta Psychiatr Scand* **89**: 81–7.

Kasanin J. (1933) The acute schizoaffective psychoses. *Am J Psychiatry* **13**: 97–126.

Kraepaelin E. (1893) *Psychiatrie. 4th Edn.* (Leipzig: Barth).

Levinson DF, Umapathy C, Musthaq M. (1999) Treatment of schizoaffective disorders and schizophrenia with mood symptoms. *Am J Psychiatry* **156**: 1138–48.

Meltzer HY, Okayli G. (1995) Reduction of suicidality during clozapine treatment of neuroleptic resistant schizophrenia: impact on risk-benefit assessment. *Am J Psychiatry* **152**: 183–90.

Penn DL, Hope DA, Spaulding W, Kucera J. (1994) Social anxiety in schizophrenia. *Schizophrenia Res* **11**: 277–84.

Siris SG. (1991) Diagnosis of secondary depression in schizophrenia: implications for DSM-IV. *Schizophrenia Bull* **17**: 75–98.

Siris SG. (1995) Depression and schizophrenia. In: (Hirsch SR, Weinberger DR, eds) *Schizophrenia.* (Blackwell Science: Oxford: 128–45.)

Siris SG. (2000) Depression in schizophrenia: prespective in the era of 'atypical' antipsychotic agents. *Am J Psychiatry* **157**: 1379–89.

Stengel E. (1945) A study of some clinical aspects of the relationship between obsessional neurosis and psychotic reaction types. *J Ment Sci* **91**: 166–87.

Tollefson GD, Sanger TM, Lu Y, Thieme ME. (1998) Depressive signs and symptoms in schizophrenia: a prospective blinded trial of olanzapine and haloperidol. *Arch Gen Psychiatry* **55**: 250–8.

Van Putten T, May PRA. (1978) 'Akinetic depression' in schizophrenia. *Arch Gen Psychiatry* **35**: 1101–7.

Wallace CJ, Nelson CJ, Liberman RP et al. (1980) A review and critique of social skills training with schizophrenic patients. *Schizophrenia Bull* **6**: 42–63.

Zohar J, Kaplan Z, Benjamin J (1993) Clomipramine treatment of obsessive–compulsive symptomatology in schizophrenic patients. *J Clin Psychiatry* **54**: 385–8.

chapter 6

Substance abuse comorbidity in schizophrenia

Wynne James and David Castle

Research over the past 30 years has explored the prevalence and possible causes of substance misuse among people with schizophrenia, as well as highlighting some of the complications that can occur as a consequence. While these studies have significantly improved the understanding of the complex interplay between drug misuse and schizophrenia, only a small number of research studies have evaluated treatment interventions aimed at improving outcomes for this group.

This chapter discusses a number of important considerations essential for a clear understanding of the relationship between substance misuse and schizophrenia; these include prevalence, impact on the course of the illness, clinical implications and reasons for use. Studies addressing substance use in schizophrenia are reviewed, a brief overview of a novel psychosocial treatment programme aimed at directly dealing with substance abuse in this population is given, and medication strategies for people with schizophrenia and substance abuse are outlined.

It should be noted that cigarette smoking and caffeine abuse are also very common amongst people with schizophrenia (e.g. Jablensky et al, 2000), and these carry their own health risks. In this chapter, however, only alcohol and illicit substances are considered.

Prevalence of substance abuse

The prevalence of substance abuse among people with schizophrenia attracts considerable attention from service providers and researchers (Mueser et al, 2000). However, studies in this area frequently suffer from a number of shortcomings, notably with respect to defining 'caseness'. This problem arises from the lack of standardized instruments used to determine diagnoses and for indexing degrees of substance use. Poor sampling procedures contribute by overrepresenting patients from urban areas, where substance use is often more prevalent. Berkson's bias also operates, in that the effect of coming to the attention of services consequent upon each individual disorder is additive and so results in higher rates of comorbidity than in non-clinical samples (Fowler et al, 1998).

There is also considerable variability in reported prevalence rates with respect to the different groups of drugs used, a fact easily obscured by the use of umbrella terms such as 'drug abuse'. Different drugs have different physical and psychological consequences, and any evaluation regarding treatment interventions should be as specific as possible about what works best with respect to each individual drug class. Finally, any results regarding prevalence rates are strongly influenced by local trends, and the legal and social status of particular drugs in particular settings, making the generalizability of results questionable. The weaknesses of prevalence studies are summarized in Box 6.1.

Box 6.1 Summary of weaknesses of prevalence studies of substance abuse in schizophrenia.

Lack of standardized instruments used to determine diagnosis
No consensus about 'caseness'
Research sampling procedures likely to reflect bias
Berkson's bias
Poor distinction between various degrees of substance use
Varying global patterns of drug use

These issues aside, there is now a general consensus that substance use disorders occur more frequently among people with schizophrenia than in the general population. In a recent review, Cantor-Graae et al (2001) found 47 studies recording prevalence of substance abuse/dependence amongst people with a psychotic illness since 1990. Of these, 37 were conducted in North America, eight in Europe, and one each in Australia and Africa. Rates of use varied widely, dependent upon the criteria applied and the setting, but lifetime rates for abuse of 'any substance' tended to aggregate at around 40–60%. Alcohol and cannabis were the leading drugs in all settings; other drugs of abuse varied by setting. Poly-drug abuse is also a feature of this clinical group; e.g. Spencer et al (2002), in an Australian sample, found that around 50% of psychosis patients regularly used more than one substance.

Community studies give a less biased assessment of rates of substance use and allow comparison with controls who do not have a mental illness. Perhaps the most frequently cited community prevalence study of mental disorders, the US Epidemiological Catchment Area Survey (ECA; Regier et al, 1990), estimated that 47% of people with schizophrenia also met criteria for lifetime substance abuse or dependence. Around one third of this group had a substance abuse disorder in the previous 6 months (Mueser at al, 1995); the lifetime rate of substance abuse in controls was around 17%. In the recent Australian Study on Low Prevalence [psychotic] Disorders (Jablensky et al, 2000), lifetime rates of substance abuse or dependence amongst people with psychotic disorders were 38.7% for males and 17.0% for females (compared with 9.4 and 3.7%, respectively, in the general population) for alcohol, and 36.3% of men and 15.7% of women (compared to 3.1 and 1.3% 12-month prevalence in the general population) for illicit substances. The most commonly abused illicit substance was cannabis, followed by amphetamines, LSD, heroin and tranquillizers; 19.1% of the sample were using more than one drug; 12% of the sample had wanted, but felt unable, to stop or cut down their substance use.

Impact of substance abuse on the course of schizophrenia

Whilst it has been shown in a number of studies that substance abuse often precedes the onset of psychotic symptoms in psychotic disorders (Linszen et al, 1994; Caspari, 1999), this does not imply causality; indeed, whether such substances can actually cause disorders such as schizophrenia is open to considerable conjecture (see Castle and Ames, 1996). What is generally accepted is that use of substances such as cannabis can precipitate psychotic episodes in vulnerable individuals (Castle and Ames, 1996). Furthermore, most studies [but not all – e.g. see Cantor-Graae et al (2001)] report that substance abuse among people with psychotic disorders tends to be associated with a poorer illness trajectory. Substance abuse has been identified as a significant factor in contributing to an increase in the number of psychotic symptoms and relapses. This is especially so with respect to patients who abuse psychotogenic drugs such as cannabis and cocaine, with heavier use of these drugs correlating with a worse symptom profile (Dixon, 1999). It is also the case that patients with psychotic disorders who abuse substances generally have a better longitudinal course than non-using counterparts if they stop using (see Krystal et al, 1999). This again reinforces the need to assist people with a vulnerability to psychotic illnesses to gain control of, and limit, their use of alcohol and illicit substances.

Clinical implications of substance abuse

Substance abuse is positively correlated with poor **treatment adherence** and as a result is a contributing factor to the worse outcome observed in this clinical group (Owen et al, 1996). Another major cause for concern among service providers and clinicians is **violence**. A number of studies have identified substance abuse as a significant risk factor for violence in people with psychotic disorders (RachBeisel et al, 1999). Cuffel et al (1994) found that poly-substance abuse among this group was associated with a significant increase in the likelihood of violent behaviours, including threats, destruction of property, assault and suicide.

Prevalence rates for **blood-borne viruses** such as HIV are higher among people with psychotic disorders complicated by substance abuse (Carey et al, 1995). These findings underscore the requirement for ongoing health education strategies that are sensitive to the needs of specific groups. Harm-reduction interventions should be a priority for clients involved in high-risk activities such as intravenous drug use and clinicians should be proactive in delivering them.

Homelessness is another significant problem for this group (Drake et al, 1991), which, in turn, complicates ongoing management by treatment services. Not surprisingly, rates of psychiatric **hospitalization** are high among people with substance abuse comorbidity (Bartels et al, 1993), and as inpatient psychiatric services remain an expensive and limited resource this is a major concern for service providers.

Thus, it is clear that the use of alcohol and illicit substances has a negative impact on people with psychotic disorders. Box 6.2 summarizes these parameters. It is important to develop more effective methods of engaging such individuals in treatments that address their substance use.

Motivations for substance use

Gaining a better understanding of motivations for substance use is an important first step in developing more effective treatments for people

---

Box 6.2 Clinical implications of substance abuse in schizophrenia.

An increase in positive symptoms
Difficulty in maintaining stable housing
Money management problems
Blood-borne virus risk behaviour
Higher rates of violent behaviour
Higher rates of hospitalization

with psychotic disorders. This aspect of substance use is still poorly understood. The notion of self-medication was for many years the predominant theory used to explain the higher rates of substance abuse among people with psychotic disorders (Siegfried, 1998). This hypothesis suggests that substance abuse is an attempt by the individual to deal with symptoms of their illness, or to counteract some of the unwanted side effects attributed to psychiatric medications. While this theory cannot be discounted, recent studies have identified a number of other factors involved in the aetiology of substance abuse among people with psychotic illnesses (see Box 6.3).

In a study investigating motivations for use in people with psychosis (mainly schizophrenia), Spencer et al (2002) found that, while there was some evidence to confirm the notion of self-medication, many respondents attributed their substance use to the same motivations as those given by the general population. Thus, these subjects reported that their substance use was driven by social motives such as conformity and acceptance, and was seen as a way of enhancing mood and improving social interaction. Another consideration lending support to these findings is that, as stated above, drug use among this group generally reflects local community drug trends, rather than there being a specific correlation between certain symptoms or side effects and use of certain drugs of

---

Box 6.3 Reasons for substance abuse by people with schizophrenia.

Self-medication: the relief of distressing symptoms and/or side effects of medication
Enhancement: 'to make you feel good'
Social motives: 'it's what others do'
Coping with unpleasant affect: 'to forget your worries'
Conformity: 'not to be left out'
Acceptance: 'to be liked'
Changing moral attitudes towards drugs use
Increased availability
Community psychiatric care

abuse (Dixon, 1999). It is probable that a number of factors contribute to the high rate of substance abuse in people with psychotic disorders and that many of these factors are the same as those mediating abuse in patients without such disorders. Mueser et al (1998), for example, have suggested a multifactorial model with antisocial personality disorder and supersensitivity to substances of abuse being contributory factors. The challenge for the field is to establish treatments that are responsive to these motivations for use, such that patients can be engaged in a treatment that is relevant and responsive to their particular makeup and situation.

Treatments for substance use in psychosis

Whilst substance use is an acknowledged problem in mental health settings, it often goes undetected and thus untreated. Part of the reason for this is the traditional dichotomy between substance misuse and mental health services, and also the lack of acceptable and well-validated treatments (Drake et al, 1998). It is widely acknowledged that treatments for substance use and mental health comorbidity are preferably developed as part of an integrated treatment approach; this implies incorporating aspects from both mental health and substance abuse treatments, and these being delivered simultaneously by the same personnel (Ley et al, 2001). Thus, treatments should be nested in clinical practice settings and involve collaboration among different health professionals. This is often not the case in current clinical practice and services are more often that not polarized, such that the substance-using person with a psychotic illness 'falls between the cracks'.

Furthermore, there remains a major deficit in terms of defining the most effective content, shape and form of interventions which will assist people with substance use comorbidity to control their substance use. Drake et al (1998) have reviewed published studies in this area: they found 36 relevant studies, including patients with an array of psychiatric disorders. Only four of the 36 studies assessed **specific treatment groups** as an addition to existing services: all had small numbers of participants and a substantial drop-out rate, none incorporated a motivational element, none were controlled and none used established outcome measures. Nine further studies evaluated **intensive integrated treatments**, which were multifaceted and very labour intensive (several hours per day for weeks to months); again, there was a substantial drop-out, making formal evaluation difficult. A further 13 studies (four controlled) were part of the US **Community Support Program (CSP)**, with a total of 1157 participants. These studies used heterogeneous interventions, which were often modified as they were being delivered, making it impossible to assess which elements were effective. Few standardized measures were used and statistical analyses were limited. Finally, 10 studies (four controlled) assessed **comprehensive integrated services**; again, the interventions were multifaceted, including intensive case management, assertive outreach and individual counselling, precluding assessment of effective elements.

Thus, existing studies have notable methodological flaws, often entail very time-consuming and therapist-intensive interventions, and give little indication of precisely which elements of the intervention are effective (or not). Many of the strategies described are not practical to implement outside research settings and do not appear to be generalizable either across treatment settings (e.g. mental health and non-government services; early episode and chronic rehabilitation settings) or to patients at different stages of their illness (e.g. early episode, chronic). Furthermore, they are generally not informed by assessment of the motivations for use by the particular individual, preventing tailoring of the intervention to the individual patient. Finally, very few studies have undertaken adequate rigorous scientific evaluation of the intervention, using a controlled experimental design and validated assessment instruments.

Psychosocial treatments

Despite the flaws in the literature on treatment interventions for substance use in schizophrenia, there is growing consensus about what features such interventions should contain (Drake and Mueser, 2000)

Box 6.4 Content of psychosocial treatment interventions for
substance abuse in schizophrenia.*

Interventions congruent with readiness to change
Not abstinence focused
Psychoeducation
Harm-reduction interventions
Motivation enhancement strategies
Relapse-prevention strategies
Peer orientated
Offers links to other supportive agencies

*Based on Drake and Mueser (2000).

(see Box 6.4). Provided here is an outline of a group psychosocial treatment interventions for substance abuse in schizophrenia that incorpo-
rate many of these elements (Castle et al, 2002). This example illustrates
many of the features currently advocated in the literature and draws
from work undertaken by, amongst others, Marlatt and Gordon (1985),
Miller and Rollnick (1991), Zeidonis and Fisher (1994), Kavanagh (1995),
Graham (1998) and Spencer et al (2002).

The intervention is delivered in an outpatient setting over a 6–8 week
period and utilizes peer support, motivational enhancement strategies,
relapse prevention and harm minimization approaches. It is available as
an adjunct to existing multidisciplinary case management services and is
for people who have a psychotic condition and who also use drugs. The
group was designed with the following broad aims:

• to establish motivations for use, and tailor intervention strategies for
  individuals on the basis of these motivations;
• to provide a forum for participants to discuss the pros and cons of
  drug use;
• to provide up-to-date information to enable participants to make
  informed choices;

- to enhance motivation to reduce drug use or to minimize the associated problems;
- to encourage participants to develop ways of managing their symptoms, relieving boredom or engaging in social activities without relying on drugs.

Importantly, there is the capacity to tailor the precise elements of the intervention to individuals within the group, based on and responsive to the factors that motivate their use of substances. This is accomplished through both exercises and examples used in the groups themselves, as well as being incorporated into the homework exercises that each participant is expected to complete. The group is divided into five modules, which can be completed in one or two sessions each. A more detailed description can be found at www.mindbodylife.com.au.

Pharmacological strategies

Another element of treatment for comorbid substance use in schizophrenia is medication. Krystal et al (1999) have provided a useful guide to pharmacotherapy of such patients. They detail the importance of optimal treatment of symptoms and prevention of side effects to counter the self-medication component of motivation for substance use. Their suggested strategies are detailed in Table 6.1.

Krystal et al (1999) also point out the potential for atypical antipsychotics (and clozapine in particular) to be associated with lower rates of substance misuse. They conjectured that this might be mediated by the particular receptor-binding profile of such agents, e.g. the blockade of serotonin $5HT_2$ receptors (potentially decreasing impulsivity), and the relative tenacity for dopamine D1 and D4 receptors (perhaps diminishing novelty seeking behaviours). Another consideration is the use of anti-addiction agents such as naltrexone and acamprosate, but the literature is limited with respect to their use in schizophrenia patients. Disulfiram may have a limited role in people with schizophrenia, but compliance is often erratic and it can exacerbate psychotic symptoms (see Krystal et al, 1999).

Table 6.1 Medication strategies to reduce self-medication with non-prescribed substances by people with schizophrenia*

Symptom/side effect	Therapeutic intervention
Extrapyramidal side effects	Lower dose of typical antipsychotic Use atypical antipsychotic
Persistent positive symptoms	Optimize control; consider clozapine
Enduring negative symptoms	Ensure not secondary to typical antipsychotic, depression, positive symptoms Consider atypical agent, notably clozapine
Emotional distress	Antidepressant/benzodiazepine Mood stabilizer Atypical antipsychotic
Cognitive dysfunction	Lower dose of typical antipsychotic Reduce benzodiazepines and anticholinergics Switch to atypical agent

*Adapted from Krystal et al (1999).

Conclusions

Substance abuse comorbidity in schizophrenia is a major problem both in terms of prevalence and the potential negative impact on illness course. Much needs to be done to enhance current understanding of what drives this comorbidity and to refine therapeutic interventions.

References

Arndt S, Tyrrell G, Flaum M et al. (1992) Comorbidity of substance abuse and schizophrenia: the role of premorbid adjustment. *Psychol Med* **22**: 379–88.

Bartels S, Teague G, Drake R et al. (1993) Substance abuse in schizophrenia: service utilisation and costs. *J Nerv Ment Dis* **181**: 227–32.

Cantor-Graae E, Nordstrom LG, McNeil TF. (2001) Substance abuse in schizophrenia: a review of the literature and a study of correlates in Sweden. *Schizophrenia Res* **48**: 69–82.

Carey M, Weinhardt L, Carey K. (1995) Prevalence of infection with HIV among the seriously mentally ill: review of research and implications for practice. *Prof Psychol: Res Prac* **26**: 262–8.

Caspari D. (1999) Cannabis and schizophrenia: results of a follow-up study. *Eur Arch Psychiatry Clin Neurosci* **249**: 45–9.

Castle DJ, Ames FR. (1996) Cannabis and the brain. *Aust NZ J Psychiatry* **30**: 179–83.

Castle D, James W, Koh G et al. (2002) Substance use in schizophrenia: why do people use, and what can we do about it? *Schizophrenia Res* **53**: 223 (abstract).

Cuffel B J, Shunway M, Chouljian T L, MacDonald T. (1994) A longitudinal study of substance use and community violence in schizophrenia. *J Nerv Ment Dis* **182**: 704–8.

Dixon L. (1999) Dual diagnosis of substance abuse in schizophrenia: prevalence and impact on outcomes. *Schizophrenia Res* **35**: 93–100.

Drake R, Antosca L, Noordsy D et al. (1991) New Hampshire's specialised services for the dually diagnosed. *New Direct Ment Health Serv* **50**: 57–67.

Drake RE, Mercer-McFadden C, Mueser KT et al. (1998) Review of integrated mental health and substance abuse treatment for patients with dual disorders. *Schizophrenia Bull* **24**: 105–18.

Drake R, Mueser K. (2000) Psychosocial approaches to dual diagnosis. *Schizophrenia Bull* **26**: 105–18.

Fowler I, Carr V, Carter N et al. (1998) Patterns of current and lifetime substance use in schizophrenia. *Schizophrenia Bull* **24**: 443–5.

Galanter M, Egelko S, De Leon G et al. (1992) Crack/cocaine abusers in the general hospital: assessment and initiation of care. *Am J Psychiatry* **149**: 810–15.

Graham HL. (1998) The role of dysfunctional beliefs in individuals who experience psychosis and use substances: implications for cognitive therapy and medication adherence. *Behav Cognit Psychother* **26**: 193–208.

Huxley N, Rendall M, Sederer L et al. (2000) Psychosocial treatments in schizophrenia: a review of the past 20 years. *J Nerv Ment Dis* **188**: 187–201.

Jablensky A, McGrath JJ, Herrman H et al. (2000) Psychotic disorders in urban areas: an overview of the Study on Low Prevalence Disorders. *Aust NZ J Psychiatry* **34**: 221–36.

Kavanagh D. (1995) An intervention for substance abuse in schizophrenia. *Behav Change* **12**: 20–30.

Krystal JH, D'Souza CD, Madonick S, Petrakis IL. (1999) Toward a rational pharmacotherapy of comorbid substance abuse in schizophrenic patients. *Schizophrenia Res* **35**: S35–S49.

Ley A, McLaren S, Siegfried N. (2001) Treatment programmes for people with both severe mental illness and substance misuse (Cochrane Review). *The Cochrane Library, Issue 1*. (Update software: Oxford, UK.)

Linszen DH, Dingemans PM, Lenior ME. (1994) Cannabis abuse and the course of recent-onset schizophrenic disorders. *Arch Gen Psychiatry* **51**: 273–9.

Marlatt G, Gordon J. (1985) *Relapse Prevention: Maintenance Strategies in the Treatment of Addictive Behaviours*. (Guildford Press: New York.)

Miller W, Rollnick S. (1991) *Motivational Interviewing: Preparing People to Change Addictive Behaviour*. (Guildford Press: New York.)

Mueser KT, Bennet M, Kushner MG. (1995) Epidemiology of substance use disorders among people with chronic mental illness. In: (Lehman AF, Dixon LB, eds) *Double Jeopardy: Chronic Mental Illness and Substance Use Disorders*. (Harwood Academic Publishers: Switzerland.)

Mueser KT, Drake RE, Wallach MA. (1998) Dual diagnosis: a review of etiological theories. *Addict Behav* **23**: 717–34.

Mueser KT, Yarnold PR, Levinson DF et al. (1990) Prevalence of substance abuse in schizophrenia: demographic and clinical correlates. *Schizophrenia Bull* **16**: 31–56.

Mueser K, Yarnold P, Rosenberg S et al. (2000) Substance use disorder in hospitalised severely mentally ill psychiatric patients: prevalence, correlates and sub groups. *Schizophrenia Bull* **26**: 179–92.

Owen R, Fischer E, Booth B et al. (1996) Medication noncompliance and substance abuse among patients with schizophrenia. *Psychiatr Serv* **47**: 853–8.

RachBeisel J, Scott J, Dixon L. (1999) Co-occurring severe mental illness and substance use disorders: a review of recent research. *Psychiatr Serv* **50**: 1427–33.

Regier D, Farmer N, Rae D et al. (1990) Comorbidity of mental disorders with alcohol and other drug abuse. *J Am Med Ass* **264**: 2511–18.

Siegfried N (1998) A review of comorbidity: major mental illness and problematic substance use. *Aust NZ J Psychiatry* **32**: 707–17.

Spencer C, Castle D, Michie P. (2002) An examination of the validity of a motivational model for understanding substance use among individuals with psychotic disorders. *Schizophrenia Bull* (in press).

Ziedonis D, Fisher W. (1994) Assessment and treatment of comorbid substance abuse in individuals with schizophrenia. *Psychiatr Ann* **24**: 477–83.

chapter 7

Management of acute arousal in psychosis

David Castle and Deirdre Alderton

This chapter outlines an approach to the management of acute arousal in psychosis. It should be recognized at the outset that there are many different reasons for people with psychotic illnesses to become acutely aroused and potentially violent to themselves or others. The management of such scenarios requires an evaluation of the factors that might be contributing and, where possible, early intervention aimed at diffusing the situation prior to dangerous escalation.

'Organic' causes of acute arousal

One often missed cause of acute arousal in psychosis is the intercession of 'organic' factors, including head injury, metabolic and endocrine disturbances, and epilepsy. The patient might be experiencing an organic delirium, resulting in confusion, fear and subsequent aggression. Intoxication with alcohol and illicit substances should be considered; withdrawal states (e.g. delirium tremens) might also be operating. Prescribed medications can also play a part here, e.g. anticholinergic delirium associated with agents such as chlorpromazine or benztropine, and withdrawal states associated with benzodiazepines. Recognition and treatment of the delirium is crucial in such cases, and merely administering further medications can compound rather than resolve the problem.

Delirium usually has an acute or subacute onset and a fluctuating course. The clinical features include (see Meagher, 2001a):

- impaired attention;
- disorientation in time, place and person;
- fluctuating concentration/attention span;
- rambling speech;
- emotional lability;
- worsening towards evening;
- visual hallucinations.

The management of delirium has been reviewed by Meagher (2001b), and includes identification and treatment of the underlying cause, ensuring safety of the individual and their environment, and optimizing environmental stimulation. Medications used in delirium should not be ones that might worsen the patient's mental state. In particular, anti-psychotics with potent central anticholinergic properties (e.g. chlorpro-mazine) should probably be avoided. Haloperidol is widely used in clinical practice, in doses of 1–2 mg orally, intramuscularly or intra-venously, depending on the clinical state; it is repeatable after 30 minutes if not initially effective (Meagher, 2001b). A role for the atypical antipsychotics will almost certainly evolve, given their benign side-effect profile and lack of negative impact on cognition. Open case series of olanzapine (5–10 mg) and risperidone (1.5–4 mg) have reported their successful use in delirium, but controlled trials are required (see Meagher, 2001b). Benzodiazepines such as lorazepam (2–4 mg orally, or parenterally, every 4 hours) are particularly useful in deliria related to alcohol and other substances (Meagher, 2001b), but can aggravate delir-ium and should be used with caution; respiratory function should be monitored, particularly with parenteral use.

Acute arousal in psychosis

In the absence of delirium, patients with psychotic disorders do have a propensity to acute arousal under certain circumstances. In schizophrenia, the arousal is often mediated by fear, as the patient may feel persecuted or believe he/she is being followed and spied upon; thus, the intervention of the police or mental health services can compound matters, and result in desperate acts of self-protection. In mania, the picture is different, with irritability and explosiveness often in response to apparently trivial events, or grandiose dismissiveness.

It is as well to recognize such factors, so that initial management does not serve to escalate matters. One should also be aware of those parameters associated with aggression in people with psychosis, as outlined in Box 7.1. Past aggression is probably the most powerful of all these predictors.

Signs of arousal

Clinicians will come to recognize certain factors that are markers or predictors of imminent aggression in people with psychosis. These include: pacing, agitation, angry gestures, closing of personal space, raised angry voice and shouting. Verbal threats should always be taken seriously; one should be particularly wary if the patient is making specific threats towards a particular person and consider that person withdrawing from the situation.

There is a gradation of acute arousal from mild through moderate to severe. A useful approach is to grade the level of arousal using a

Box 7.1 Predictors of aggression in psychosis.

Young men
History of sociopathy/forensic history
Delirium, head injury
Alcohol intoxication
Illicit substance use
Psychosis, expressly if persecutory beliefs, command hallucinations
Past aggression/violence

Table 7.1 Acute arousal scale (based on the Patient Arousal Rating Scale, Fremantle Hospital & Health Service)*

Grade of arousal	Severity and symptoms of arousal
5	Highly aroused, violent towards self, others or property
4	Highly aroused and possibly distressed or fearful
3	Moderately aroused, agitated, becoming more vocal and unreasonable or hostile
2	Mildly aroused, pacing, still willing to talk reasonably
1	Settled, minimal agitation
0	Asleep or unconscious

*Symptoms of arousal include: noisy, distressed, agitated, behavioural disturbance (increased motor activity, intrusive, disinhibited), verbally abusive, physically abusive (to self, others or property), fearful.

standardized scale, such as that shown in Table 7.1. The virtue of this is that all staff can be using the same benchmarks, making assessment and communication easier, as well as guiding interventions and monitoring efficacy of each particular intervention.

Managing acute arousal: non-pharmacological strategies

It is important to ensure that staff are well informed and feel safe – a fearful patient will be reassured by the sense that staff are calm and know what they are doing. It is crucial that consistent messages are given to the patient, so it is best to have a single nominated staff member who does the talking; other attendant staff should be briefed as to what signal or words might indicate that physical restraint should be implemented.

If possible, the patient should be taken into an unstimulating environment, away from other patients, but staff should ensure that an exit can be accessed easily. Support staff should be close by, but unobtrusive. Anything that might be used as a weapon (e.g. pens, pagers, mobile phones) should be removed. The nominated staff member should talk in an even voice and not raise it. Speech should be slow and clear, other people present should be introduced, and everything that is going on should be explained. Sudden movements should be avoided. The patient should be reassured that the staff want to help him/her, and will try to work with them towards a mutually acceptable outcome (Stevenson, 1991).

If **physical restraint** is required, then sufficient support staff should be close by and know what their roles will be. Security personnel or the police should be called in where indicated. If possible, tasks for the restraint should be allocated ahead of time (e.g. arms, legs, head) and a key word signalling the restraint to designated staff. Medications intended for administration should be drawn up in advance and the person to administer them selected. The patient should be talked to throughout, offering reassurance and explanation, and trying to obtain cooperation. Staff should be debriefed afterwards (Brown, 1998).

The use of **seclusion** is somewhat controversial. It has been defined as 'placement of a patient, alone, in a specially designated lockable room from which he or she can be observed through a window' (Kirkpatrick, 1989). Benefits of seclusion include: control and safety for the individual, other patients and staff; 'time out' in a low-stimulus environment; a way of avoiding excessive use of medication. There are downsides, including the potential for perception of seclusion as punitive or a violation of patient's rights (see Wynaden et al, 2001). On balance, the judicious use of seclusion can be a safe and effective adjunct to the management of the acutely aroused patient, but its use should be carefully monitored.

Managing acute arousal: pharmacological strategies

There is a general lack of consensus regarding the pharmacological management of acute arousal in psychosis (Cunnane, 1994), though recent attempts have been made to establish expert consensus; the interested reader is referred to the guidelines by Allen et al (2001). Most clinicians would agree that high doses or cumulative doses of antipsychotics should be avoided where possible, not least because of the risk of sudden death from cardiac dysrhythmias. Also, one is aiming for rapid tranquillization rather than rapid neuroleptization, and should be aware that antipsychotic effects lag days or weeks behind tranquillizing effects (Macpherson et al, 1996).

Presented here are guidelines that have been modified and refined with serial clinical audits. Although effective in the vast majority of cases, they are only guidelines and can be modified in particular clinical situations. For example, good response to a particular agent in the past would support its use again, whilst benzodiazepines, which cause respiratory depression, should probably be avoided in patients with severe respiratory problems. Care should be taken with patients who have had an adverse reaction to an agent in the past; a history of neuroleptic malignant syndrome is of particular concern. Finally, it should be noted that the use of intravenous medication is not advocated, largely because of the potential for respiratory depression and arrest with its use; however, the intravenous route might be justified in certain clinical scenarios.

Any pharmacological intervention for acute arousal should be tailored to the particular clinical situation and the efficacy monitored closely. Thus, the use of a scale such as that shown in Table 7.1 can guide the intervention and ensure consistency of approach. Figure 7.1 shows an algorithmic approach to the management of acute arousal in psychosis, with interventions graded according to the degree of arousal.

Ideally, the patient should be offered oral medication in the first instance, and consent should be attempted for any intervention. If

STEP 1. (Arousal level 2–3)
Mildly aroused, pacing, still
willing to talk reasonably
Moderately aroused, agitated,
becoming more vocal,
unreasonable or hostile

STEP 2. (Arousal level 3–4)
Moderately aroused, agitated,
becoming more vocal,
unreasonable or hostile
Highly aroused, possibly
distressed and fearful

STEP 3. (Arousal level 4–5)
Refusing oral medication
Moderately aroused, agitated,
becoming more vocal,
unreasonable or hostile
Highly aroused, possibly
distressed and fearful, violent
towards self, others or
property

ORAL

ORAL

INTRAMUSCULAR

Lorazepam
1 mg or 2.5 mg

Review after 60 minutes,
repeat if necessary

If still ineffective consider Step 2

(If sedation required)

Chlorpromazine
100 mg or 200 mg

(atypical option:
olanzapine 10 mg)

Review after 60 minutes,
repeat if necessary

May be given with lorazepam
1 mg or 2.5 mg for extra
anxiolytic/sedative effects

Haloperidol 5 mg or 10 mg, or
droperidol 10 mg or 20 mg

(atypical option:
olanzapine 10 mg)

May be given with lorazepam
1 mg or 2.5 mg for extra
anxiolytic/sedative effects

(If a more rapid but shorter
effect is required use
midazolam 0.1 mg/kg)

Review after 30 minutes,
repeat if necessary

OR

Precautions

Lower doses should be
considered in the elderly,
patients with low body weight,
dehydration or no previous
exposure to antipsychotic
medications

Monitor respiratory function
when benzodiazepines are
ministered parenterally

Monitor postural blood
pressure after each dose

Haloperidol 5 mg or 10 mg, or
zuclopenthixol 10–25 mg

(atypical option:
risperidone 2 mg)

Review after 60 minutes,
repeat if necessary

May be given with lorazepam
1 mg or 2.5 mg for extra
anxiolytic/sedative effects

If still ineffective consider Step 3

Cautions

• EPSEs' should be
  monitored and treated

• Benztropine 2 mg IM or IV
  may be required for acute
  dystonias
  (max 6 mg/24 hours)

• Anticholinergic agents NOT
  to be used routinely but on
  an as-required basis

Figure 7.1 Guidelines for the management of acute arousal and agitation in psychosis. EPSE, extrapyramidal side effects; IM, intramuscularly; IV, intravenously.

restraint and forced injection is required, certain criteria need to be met, including that the patient be detained under the local Mental Health Act (a single restraint and forced medication may be permissible under duty of care, but this should be done only under exceptional circumstances). It should be noted that in patients experiencing their first episode of psychosis (i.e. neuroleptic naïve), in the elderly, in those with medical conditions or in those with a history of adverse reactions to antipsychotics, doses should be lowered.

The administration of medication in this setting should be closely monitored and the efficacy or otherwise of particular interventions assessed at set time periods, which should be stipulated by the prescribing doctor (usually 30 minutes for intramuscular medications and 60 minutes for oral medication). A proforma for the documentation of such information is shown in Figure 7.2. This also allows a rapid appraisal of total medication use over a period of time.

It should also be noted that the algorithm promotes benzodiazepines and typical antipsychotics, with atypical antipsychotics as optional. As discussed below, atypicals might well come to supersede typicals in the acute arousal scenario, but the current evidence base is small and clinical experience with parenteral atypicals is limited.

The problems associated with typical antipsychotics in the acute setting include cardiac conduction problems, postural hypotension, acute dystonias, akathisia and neuroleptic malignant syndrome. Benzodiazepines can cause disinhibition and even exacerbation of mania in some individuals. Awareness of these potential outcomes should lead to the monitoring of the patient in terms of mental state, extrapyramidal side effects, and pulse rate and blood pressure. Serial electrocardiograms and blood tests, including creatine phosphokinase (CPK) levels (see Chapter 1), should be performed where clinically indicated, and whenever high cumulative doses of antipsychotic agents have been administered.

Atypical antipsychotics

The role of the atypical antipsychotics (e.g. risperidone, olanzapine, quetiapine, ziprasidone) in the management of acute arousal has not yet been fully evaluated and has been restricted until recently by the lack of

WARD	WEIGHT (kg)	AGE	Patient's Name .... Unit No ....

Christian Name ....

Address ....

Total Number of Medication Charts ....

Chart Numbers ....

Sex .... Birth Date .... Age ....

Step 1	MEDICATION	Dose	Route	Additional Information
				Check for effect after
Date	Dr Print Name	Dr Sign		Pharm	Imprest DD

Step 2	MEDICATION	Dose	Route	Additional Information
				Check for effect after
Date	Dr Print Name	Dr Sign		Pharm	Imprest DD

Step 3	MEDICATION	Dose	Route	Additional Information
				Check for effect after
Date	Dr Print Name	Dr Sign		Pharm	Imprest DD

Step	Date	Time	1st Rating	Dose Given	Route	Nurse	Check	2nd Rating	Time	Nurse's Signature

Figure 7.2 *Agitation and arousal medication chart. Based on charts used at the Fremantle Hospital, Western Australia.*

parenteral forms of these agents. Short-acting intramuscular forms of olanzapine and ziprasidone have now been produced, and are coming into clinical use.

As outlined above, it is likely, given their relatively benign side-effect profile, that atypicals will come to be important in the management of acute arousal (see Figure 7.1). Indeed, early data suggest that oral risperidone liquid compares favourably with intramuscular haloperidol in the control of psychotic agitation (Currier and Simpson, 2000). Olanzapine is available in a quick-dissolving wafer form that is useful in the acute setting; studies comparing the use of intramuscular olanzapine with intramuscular haloperidol have demonstrated a faster onset of action with the former in the treatment of acute agitation, and a lower risk of extrapyramidal side effects (EPSE) (Wright et al, 2001). Intramuscular ziprasidone also compares favourably with haloperidol in acute arousal, and appears to be well tolerated and safe (Brook et al, 2002). The present authors are not aware of any published studies on the use of quetiapine in acute arousal but some clinicians report beneficial use in this setting, with a rapid up-titration; care needs to be taken to monitor blood pressure, as postural hypotension may occur in this context.

The role of zuclopenthixol (Clopixol Acuphase)

One particular agent has a special place in the management of acute arousal – zuclopenthixol [Clopixol Acuphase (acuphase)] (see Fenton et al, 2000; Barnes et al, 2002). This agent (not available in some countries) is essentially a short-acting depot, with an effect lasting some 24–48 hours. It is very sedating and the fact that it is relatively long-lasting means that the requirement for numerous repeated injections is reduced, relative to shorter acting agents. Ideally, acuphase should be used as a course of three to four injections, at least 24 hours apart, as detailed in Figure 7.3 and Box 7.2. The patient needs to be monitored, particularly with respect to blood pressure (it can cause profound postural hypotension) and EPSE. Acuphase should be considered a

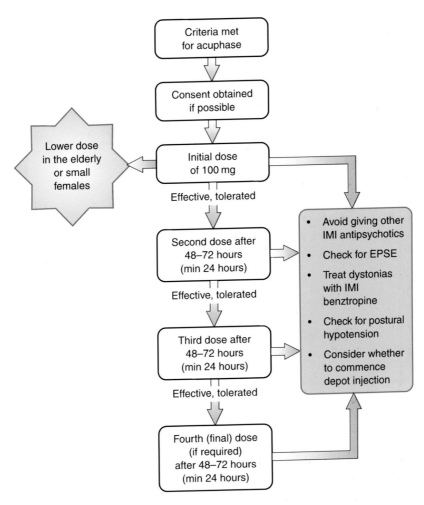

Figure 7.3 Guidelines for the use of zuclopenthixol [Clopixol Acuphase (acuphase)]. IMI, intramuscular injection; EPSE, extrapyramidal side effects. Based on Barnes et al (2002) with permission. (For prescribing guidelines, see Box 7.2)

Box 7.2 Prescribing guidelines for the use of zuclopenthixol acetate [Clopixol Acuphase (acuphase)].

Initial treatment of **acute arousal** and **agitation** in psychosis is described in Figure 7.1. Acuphase should be considered a treatment rather than an emergency intervention for acute arousal and an effort should be made, where feasible, to obtain verbal informed consent from the patient. Acuphase should not usually be used for first-episode patients.

Suitable patients for the prescription of acuphase
- Those who have received step 3 injections as per Figure 7.1 more than once **and** have had sufficient time for the assessment of response and/or side effects to previously injected drugs (minimum 30–60 minutes) (see Figure 7.1, step 3).
- Those who have previously received acuphase and have shown a good tolerability **and** response to it.

Prescribing information for acuphase
- The standard dose is 100 mg every 48–72 hours;
- females, neuroleptic-naïve patients and the elderly may require lower than standard doses (25 or 50 mg every 48–72 hours);
- large young males may require higher than standard doses (up to 150 mg every 48–72 hours);
- a course of injections is usually prescribed (e.g. 100 mg every 48–72 hours): the maximum dose is 400 mg over 2 weeks or four injections, whichever comes first;
- at least 24 hours must elapse between acuphase injections;
- the patient should be monitored carefully for extrapyramidal side effects (EPSE), which should be treated vigorously if they occur;
- blood pressure should be monitored carefully (hypotension may occur).

Sedation effects of acuphase
- Sedation may initially be seen 15–90 minutes after injection, peaking after 8 hours;
- sedation effects may last for up to 72 hours;
- the first injection is usually the most sedating;
- acuphase may need to be given with IMI lorazepam or midazolam if immediate sedation is required (note: these drugs must be administered separately and not mixed in the same syringe);

- attempts should be made to avoid the use of other **parenteral antipsychotics** when patients are receiving a course of acuphase;
- acuphase may be mixed in the same syringe with the first dose of flupenthixol or zuclopenthixol decanoate if a depot is to be initiated.

Patients in whom caution is advised in the use of acuphase
- Those who are concurrently receiving other antipsychotics.
- Those who are sensitive to EPSE.
- Those who have pre-existing cardiac disease.

Care should be taken if the patient is struggling, as acuphase is dangerous if given into a vein.

Selection of patients suitable for treatment with acuphase
Acuphase is especially effective in the treatment of:
- aggression/arousal which is difficult to bring under control;
- relapse of chronic schizophrenia;
- manic relapse.

Adapted from Barnes et al (2002), with permission.

treatment rather than an emergency intervention *per se*, so an attempt should be made to gain consent from the patient (Fitzgerald, 1999).

Conclusions

Acute arousal is not uncommon in psychiatric settings, endangering both patients and staff. It is important to try to understand what drives the arousal and to intervene before matters escalate. If pharmacological management is required, this needs to be administered in a structured and safe manner, and the effects and side effects carefully monitored.

Acknowledgements

We wish to acknowledge the staff of the Psychiatric Intensive Care Unit and Fremantle Hospital, Western Australia, for their role in development and piloting many of the strategies suggested here.

References

Allen MH, Currier GW, Hughes DH et al. (2001) Treatment of behavioral emergencies. *Postgrad Med (Spec Rep)*, 1–88.

Barnes CW, Alderton D, Castle DJ. (2002) The development of clinical guidelines for the use of zuclopenthixol acetate. *Austr Psychiatry* **10:** 54–8.

Brook S, Walden J, Benattia I. (2002) Ziprasidone vs. halpoperidol in sequential im/oral treatment of acute schizophrenia. *Schizophrenia Res* **53:** 181.

Brown T. (1998) Psychiatric emergencies. *Adv Psychiatr Treat* **4:** 270–6.

Cunnane JG. (1994) Drug management of disturbed behaviour by psychiatrists. *Psychiatr Bull* **18:** 138–9.

Currier GW, Simpson GM. (2000) Risperidone liquid concentrate and oral lorazepam versus intramuscular haloperidol for treatment of psychotic agitation. *J Clin Psychiatry* **62:** 153–7.

Fenton M, Coutinho ESF, Campell C. (2000) Zuclopenthixol acetate in the treatment of acute schizophrenia and similar serious mental illness (Cochrane Review). *Cochrane Library, Issue 1.* (Update Software: Oxford, UK.)

Fitzgerald P. (1999) Long acting antipsychotic medication, restraint and treatment in the management of acute psychosis. *Aust NZ J Psychiatry* **33:** 660–6.

Kirkpatrick H. (1989) A descriptive study of seclusion: the unit environment, patient behaviour, and nursing interventions. *Arch Psychiatr Nursing* **3:** 3–9.

Macpherson R, Anstee B, Dix R. (1996) Guidelines for the management of acutely disturbed patients. *Adv Psychiatr Treat* **2:** 194–201.

Meagher DJ. (2001a) Delirium: the role of psychiatry. *Adv Psychiatr Treat* **7:** 433–43.

Meagher DJ. (2001b) Delirium: optimizing management. *Br Med J* **322:** 144–9.

Stevenson S. (1991) Heading off violence with verbal de-escalation. *J Psychosoc Nursing Ment Health Serv* **29:** 6–10.

Wright P, Birkett M, David S et al. (2001) Double-blind, placebo controlled comparison of intramuscular olanzapine and intramuscular haloperidol in the treatment of acute agitation in schizophrenia. *Am J Psychiatry* **158:** 1149–51.

Wynaden D, Orb A, McGowan S et al. (2001) The use of seclusion in the year 2000: what has changed? *Collegian* **8:** 19–25.

chapter 8

Promoting adherence to treatment in schizophrenia

Peter Hayward and Til Wykes

Traditionally, the term compliance has been used to refer to the degree to which a patient follows medical advice and complies with treatment recommendations. Patients who take their tablets are said to be compliant, while those who refuse or forget are called non-compliant, or are described as showing poor compliance. It has been suggested that these labels promote a one-sided view of the consultation process: the doctor offers wise and correct advice, and the sensible patient obeys without question. The term adherence has been advocated recently as suggesting a more active role for the patient, while the Royal Pharmaceutical Society of Great Britain (1997) suggest the term concordance as promoting the idea of negotiation between patient and prescriber. Ideally, the consultation process and the devising of treatment recommendations, whether they involve pharmacological, psychosocial or other types of treatment, should be a process of collaborative empiricism where the patient is treated as an equal partner. Not only is there empirical evidence that this approach leads to superior treatment outcome and greater patient satisfaction, but it respects the autonomy of the patient. How to improve adherence in practice is what will be expanded on throughout this chapter.

Factors affecting adherence

A variety of factors can either promote or undermine treatment adherence (see Box 8.1). As a rule, adherence to treatment regimes is far lower than professionals might wish, for most medical conditions. It has been suggested that around 50% of patients adhere to a variety of long-term treatment regimes, for illnesses including heart disease, asthma and AIDS. Consider for a moment the well-established rules of a healthy lifestyle: avoidance of alcohol, tobacco and fattening foods, regular exercise, low levels of stress, daily flossing of the teeth: do you always adhere to all these practices? In general, people tend to take treatment when they are in distress, while preventative treatments are often forgotten. This is, of course, especially true of patients who don't believe that they are ill but have other explanations for their problems, such as paranoid or grandiose delusions. Low intelligence quotient (IQ) and disorganized thinking may interfere with adherence, especially if medication regimes are complicated. Side effects may also be a problem, but these effects are often individual

Box 8.1 Factors affecting adherence.

The person
Cultural and family values
Experiences of illness and treatment
Support network and milieu
Personality
Psychological reactance
Intelligence
Views of illness

The treatment
Therapeutic alliance
Treatment setting
Effectiveness
Complexity
Side effects
Stigma

The illness
Delusional beliefs
Positive aspects of illness experience
Depression/anxiety
Cognitive impairment
Lack of motivation

with one patient finding a particular side effect intolerable whilst another will find it much less problematic. For example, one patient might be terribly upset by sexual dysfunction but indifferent to weight gain whereas another patient might feel the exact opposite. Patients with psychiatric conditions are more likely to adhere to long-term treatments if:

- they see benefit in them;
- the treatments are easily available and uncomplicated to take;
- they are offered in a pleasant and convenient setting by professionals who they like, and who show them respect and offer them other kinds of practical help.

Most importantly, the treatments should be effective and provide benefits that outweigh their side effects.

In addition to the factors that are outlined in Box 8.1, there are other issues, some of which are confused with treatment adherence and others which must be considered as background factors in treatment adherence. The main issues are: insight, reactance, and stigma; these are described below.

Insight

Traditionally, the term insight is used to mean the correct understanding, by the patient, of his illness. This terminology has been criticized as meaning, in practice, that insight consists of agreeing with the doctor. For many of those with long-term mental illness, their strange beliefs and experiences seem obviously true, significant and, in some cases, even life-enhancing. To perceive oneself as extraordinarily important or in intimate contact with a famous or attractive person might be seen as being very desirable; to some, even to be persecuted by enemies with strange powers might be seen as better than being completely ignored by everyone. While some sufferers may well find the belief that their experiences are just an illness as comforting, others may well prefer other types of explanation. Some measures of insight actually use treatment adherence as one part of the measure (see David, 1990), but it is important to note that having good insight does not necessarily mean that one will adhere to treatment. The opposite is also true, i.e. patients may adhere to a treatment regime whilst denying the illness for which it was prescribed.

Reactance

The concept of reactance, which has strong theoretical links with that of non-adherence, has been used for the tendency people have to react negatively to pressure and coercion; when told forcibly that they must do something, some people go along with it, while others will react in exactly the opposite way (Fogarty, 1997). Moore et al (2000) found that the degree of psychological reactance was a good predictor of treatment adherence. This would suggest that, for those high in reactance, adherence to treatment could best be achieved by a non-confrontational approach, by convincing the patient to choose freely to receive treatment. Unfortunately, many patients undergo their first experience of psychiatric treatment involuntarily, by being detained in hospital. This will often be a highly distressing experience that can result in a legacy of antagonism and resentment within that person.

Stigma

There is strong research evidence that lay people hold stigmatizing and prejudiced views about the mentally ill, and that these views discourage sufferers from seeking treatment (Hayward and Bright, 1997). The lay public seems to know relatively little about those with serious mental illness, but to see such people as bizarre, difficult and dangerous. Further, lay people often define mental illness in terms of treatment received rather than in terms of symptoms exhibited. Thus, most people will be slow to accept that they have a stigmatized condition. Labelling in this context becomes very important; it is not necessary to insist that a person accept a diagnostic label, or even a label of illness, in order to benefit from treatment. To say that a treatment may help to relieve stress or might help someone to cope better might well be more acceptable to many people, and these statements are also true. If patient and professional agree on a treatment approach, does it really matter if they disagree on the diagnostic label?

Promoting adherence

Failure to adhere to prescribed medication is one of the major causes of relapse among sufferers from severe mental illness. At the same time, a growing body of research is demonstrating that the principles of cognitive behavioural therapy (CBT) can be used successfully to promote adaptive functioning in a variety of psychiatric conditions, including schizophrenia, paranoid psychosis and other forms of serious mental illness (see Chapter 2). In spite of this, relatively little effort has been made to use CBT techniques to enhance adherence to treatment regimes. Some of the pioneers in the field of CBT for psychosis have suggested the application of CBT techniques in this area (Kingdon and Turkington, 1994; Nelson, 1997; Beck, 2001), and a few empirical trials suggest that such approaches can improve adherence and decrease relapse rates (Kemp et al, 1996, 1998; Lecompte and Pelc, 1996; Hayashi et al, 2001). However, this is not a field that has received much empirical investigation. In spite of this, the CBT approach points the way to better understanding and concordance between patient and health professional. This is because CBT is, by its very nature, a collaborative enterprise, seeking an agreed model of the difficulties to be addressed and the ways of alleviating those difficulties. In applying such an approach to patients with major mental illness or, for that matter, any condition requiring medical treatment, the goal should not be to 'get them to take their tablets' but to first create a good treatment alliance and then to persuade patients to consider various treatment options (Perkins and Repper, 1999).

As explained in Kemp et al (1996), the process of building adherence can be conceptualized as occurring in three stages. The first is to elicit the patient's concerns and problems, and then to try and understand his or her model of the root of these difficulties. Initially, a review of illness history may be useful, although it goes without saying that it is not helpful to insist that the patient has an illness. Many patients see their problems as external or due to stress or pressures of circumstance rather than as mental illness. Kingdon and Turkington's (1994) idea of the normalizing rationale can be very helpful in this situation: patients are told that their symptoms are very common and can be seen in many people under conditions of excessive stress, thus avoiding the stigma that a label of major mental illness carries. The first goal is thus to find a rationale that is acceptable to the patient, so that the idea of medication can be introduced as a possible coping strategy to deal with ongoing problems.

The second key step with any patient is to ask her to consider the advantages and disadvantages of taking medication. Most psychotropic medications have a wide variety of potential side effects, and other issues such as diagnosis and stigma may be very important for particular patients. However, most patients will also be able to pick out advantages in particular medications, ranging from improved sleep to better relationships with loved ones. To avoid reactance, as noted above, the patient must always feel that the final choice is hers. If patients choose not to take medication, it is important to maintain a good relationship, so that if she encounters future difficulties she may be open to reconsidering this decision.

A useful tool at this point can be some form of self-monitoring (Randall et al, 2002). A simple form can be developed between the patient and professional, allowing the patient to monitor his mental state and side effects. A trial period can be suggested and, when it is over, the patient will have clear evidence as to the effectiveness or otherwise of the particular medication. Formally devised instruments may be less helpful than a simple form that focuses on the patient's own self-chosen problems (see Figure 8.1).

If medication proves effective and the patient is well, then a new problem may arise – as noted above, many people find it hard to adhere to regimes of preventative medication because people are not generally motivated to take medication when they feel well. This is the third stage of building adherence: the professional should offer advice on this point and encourage the use of long-term prophylactic treatment, pointing out both the arguments in its favour and the problems that many people will encounter. However, many patients will probably stop their medication at some point and fall ill again: such an outcome does not

Feeling anxious and threatened				
Much better	A bit better	Same	A bit worse	Much worse

Poor sleep				
Much better	A bit better	Same	A bit worse	Much worse

Restlessness				
Much better	A bit better	Same	A bit worse	Much worse

Concentration				
Much better	A bit better	Same	A bit worse	Much worse

Feeling that 'the world depends on me'				
Much better	A bit better	Same	A bit less	Much less

Dry mouth				
Much better	A bit better	Same	A bit worse	Much worse

Feeling that 'the television is talking to me'				
Much more	A bit more	Same	A bit less	Much less

Tired/no energy				
Much better	A bit better	Same	A bit worse	Much worse

Figure 8.1 *Personal checklist.*

mean failure. The establishment of a good, collaborative relationship should improve long-term engagement with services for most patients. Relapse is also not an indicator that a collaborative approach to treatment adherence is not a worthwhile one. Some patients may take a considerable time to build a trusting relationship in which they can begin to explore their own decisions about treatment.

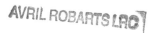

> ## Box 8.2 Enhancing adherence.
>
> **Key principles**
> Emphasize personal choice and responsibility
> Focus on patient's key concerns, personal goals, fears and worries
> Express empathy for patient's problems and dilemmas
> Support self-efficacy
>
> **Key techniques**
> Regular summarizing
> Inductive questioning to elicit patient's own concerns
> Explore pros and cons of treatment options
> Use normalizing rationale to combat stigma
> Focus on patient's own long-term goals
>
> **Approaches to avoid**
> Lecturing/preaching
> Insisting on particular diagnostic labels
> Debating with the patient
> Laying down the law

Box 8.2 provides a brief summary of some of the key elements in a collaborative approach. The present authors trust that evidence as to the benefits of this method will continue to accumulate. In any case, many sufferers and professionals find this approach to be both helpful and congenial.

References

Beck JS. (2001) A cognitive therapy approach to medication compliance. In: (Kay J, ed), *Integrated Treatment of Psychiatric Disorders*. (American Psychiatric Association: Washington DC) *Review of Psychiatry* **20**: 113–41.

Bentall RP, Jackson HF, Pilgrim D. (1988) Abandoning the concept of 'schizophrenia': some implications of validity arguments for psychological research into psychotic phenomena. *Br J Clin Psychol*, **27**: 303–24.

David AS. (1990) Insight and psychosis. *Br J Psychiatry*, **156**: 798–808.

Fogarty JS. (1997) Reactance theory and patient noncompliance. *Soc Sci Med,* **45:** 1277–88.

Hayashi N, Yamashina M, Igarashi Y, Kazamatsuri H. (2001) Improvement of patient attitude toward treatment among inpatients with schizophrenia and its related factors: controlled study of a psychological approach. *Comprehen Psychiatry* **42:** 240–6.

Hayward P, Bright JA. (1997) Stigma and mental illness: a review and critique. *J Ment Health,* **6:** 345–54.

Kemp R, David A, Hayward P. (1996) Compliance therapy: an intervention targeting insight and treatment adherence in psychotic patients. *Behav Cognit Psychother,* **24:** 331–50.

Kemp R, Kirov G, Everitt B et al. (1998) Randomised controlled trial of compliance therapy: 18–month follow-up. *Br J Psychiatry,* **172:** 413–19.

Kingdon DG, Turkington D. (1994) *Cognitive Behavioural Therapy of Schizophrenia.* (Guilford: New York).

Lecompte D, Pelc I. (1996) A cognitive–behavioral program to improve compliance with medication in patients with schizophrenia. *Int J Ment Health* **25:** 51–6.

Moore A, Sellwood W, Stirling J. (2000) Compliance and psychological reactance in schizophrenia. *Br J Clin Psychol,* **39:** 287–95.

Nelson H. (1997) *Cognitive Behavioural Therapy with Schizophrenia.* (Stanley Thornes: Cheltenham.)

Perkins RE, Repper JM. (1999) Compliance or informed choice. *J Ment Health* **8:** 117–29.

Randall F, Wood P, Day J et al. (2002) Enhancing appropriate adherence with neuroleptic medication: two contrasting approaches. In: (Morrison AP, ed), *A Casebook of Cognitive Therapy for Psychosis.* (Brunner-Routledge: Hove.)

Royal Pharmaceutical Society of Great Britain (RPSGB) (1997) *From Compliance to Concordance: Achieving Shared Goals in Medicine Taking.* (RPSGB: London.)

chapter 9

Work and recovery in schizophrenia

Morris D Bell

Working is central to the life of most healthy adults. It affects where they live, who their friends are and how they feel about themselves. Many regard their careers as expressions of their identity and part of their purpose in life. Schizophrenia is a disabling mental condition that usually disrupts a person's working life and, because it is a disorder with an onset in adolescence or early adulthood, it often interferes with the normal development of a career and worker identity. As people with schizophrenia attempt to adjust to their new reality of medications, painful refractory symptoms and profound uncertainty about their future, their efforts at recovery may be hampered by a lack of appropriate opportunity for productive activity. Since schizophrenia may attack a person's motivation and sense of purpose, as well as cause positive symptoms like paranoia and hallucinations, a person with this disorder may become discouraged about ever finding a place in the world of work.

Yet, unemployment can also cause stress. Evidence from studies on the negative effects of unemployment in the general population indicate that unemployment can lead to substance abuse, physical problems, psychiatric disorders, reduced self-esteem, loss of social contacts, alienation and apathy (Warr, 1987). Thus, unemployment and inactivity may, in fact, compound the difficulties of recovering from schizophrenia.

While it is likely that working may include challenges and stressors, working with appropriate supports and accommodations may actually reduce symptoms. For example, in one study by Bell et al (1996), people with schizophrenia reported less emotional discomfort and decreased positive symptoms as a result of working. Also, the longer they worked, the better their symptoms became. In a separate study (Bryson and Bell, 2002), people with serious mental disorders who worked reported improved quality of life. In particular, their motivation and sense of purpose improved. Those who worked longer also reported improved social relationships. These results and those of others (Mueser et al, 1997; Priebe et al, 1998; Bond et al, 2001a,b) support the favourable impact that appropriate work activity may have. Working in normal settings provides opportunities to regain a better sense of consensual reality, to be distracted from painful internal experiences and to feel a part of society. By providing structure and purpose, it may increase motivation and enhance social interactions. It is also an aspiration to the majority of people with severe mental illness.

Studies show that most people with severe mental illness would like to work and regard working as an important part of their recovery. In a recent survey, only 10% of people interviewed said that they did not want a job, although only half of those interviewed considered employment as an immediate option (Secker et al, 2001). Families also recognize and often encourage their family member to return to school or get a part-time job, although they are often unsure about how hard to push or how to help. However, despite these aspirations, the actual figures for those employed are very low. Recent estimates show that only about 15% of people with severe mental illness are employed full- or part-time (NIDRR, 1998; McQuilken et al, 2002). Institutional psychiatry has been slow to recognize the role that work can play in recovery. This is somewhat surprising given the fact that the idea of work as a treatment for the restoration of mental health has distinguished antecedents from the age of moral treatment.

A brief history of work

Moral treatment began in the early nineteenth century as an alternative to the brutal treatment of the insane that was commonly regarded as good medical practice. Moral treatment viewed the mentally ill as fellow humans, deserving of dignity, whose torments should be treated with kindness, calming influences and encouragement to redirect their thoughts in productive ways through work and education. In the USA, the Quakers founded the first asylums based upon the premises of moral treatment and, because of the reportedly good results [e.g. 58% cure rate from the Worcester asylum (Whitaker, 2002)], others soon adopted its principles. Work was regarded by these asylums to be an effective therapeutic agent that could distract patients from their psychotic preoccupations, improve self-esteem through realistic accomplishment and allow for the discharge of tension through physical activity (Brigham, 1847/1994). At the beginning of the twentieth century, most asylums continued to provide work activity – usually farming, cooking, maintenance, laundry and cottage industries – because of its putative therapeutic benefit and because it reduced operational costs. As mental institutions became overcrowded, underfunded and mismanaged, they sometimes exploited their patients, using them primarily as cheap labour without regard to their rehabilitation. Concerns about patients' rights worldwide, the introduction of antipsychotic medications and new structures for financial support in the community combined to produce the period of deinstitutionalization that has virtually eliminated the large chronic mental hospital (in Western countries at least). But, during this transition, scant attention was paid to the fact that deinstitutionalization inadvertently deprived patients of the meaningful work they had performed in the institutions. Few work programmes had been created in the community, so hospital discharge meant unemployment and inactivity.

Community services for the mentally ill have slowly improved and the needs of recovering patients have become better understood. Mental health agencies, particularly in the USA, have begun to respond to the need to provide their patients with opportunities to return to work. The USA has the largest number of work activities and the majority of these are coordinated by the US Department of Veterans Affairs (VA), which provides mental health services through a national network of medical centres and clinics. In 2001, the VA had more than 28,500 patients with severe psychiatric and substance abuse disorders enrolled on its various work programmes, earning more than $US 48 m (Mental Health Strategic Health Group, 2001, a,b). Other work programmes for the mentally disabled in the USA are provided through community mental health agencies that depend upon state funding, so commitment to these services varies from state to state. For instance, New Hampshire converted day programmes into work programmes, fully endorsing work activity as central to psychosocial rehabilitation.

What services are provided?

Work services can be described along a continuum from most to least restrictive, with sheltered workshops and enclaves being the least autonomous settings, and transitional work programmes in competitive work environments and supported employment (SE) offering the greatest autonomy. Table 9.1 shows the various categories.

All types of work programme lead to better employment than doing nothing and there is some evidence that they also lead to an increased quality of life (Bond et al, 2001a). The elements of the programmes within the categories in Table 9.1 may also vary. For instance, the schemes available in West Haven VA, Connecticut, and at the Connecticut Mental Health Center in New Haven, also include an element of cognitive retraining alongside the vocational training elements (Bell et al, 2001). Programmes may also have an eclectic approach, with integration between clubhouse models and vocational training.

Supported Employment (SE) as an evidence-based practice

For most people with severe and persistent mental disorders, SE is now endorsed as the preferred method for work rehabilitation. Eight randomized trials and three quasi-experimental studies support the generalizability of SE across a broad range of clients and settings, so that SE is regarded

Table 9.1 Types of work service

Work service	Description	Comment
Vocational counselling and training	Brokered training services in specific job skills. Guided job search based on interests and abilities	Insensitive to special needs and presumes that job success will come from job skills and counselling
Prevocational training	Small tasks performed to teach good work behaviours	Little responsibility, not in community, no pay
Sheltered workshop	Small manufacturing and assembly: piecework and little variety of work. Co-workers are similarly disabled	Feels safe but no community interaction. Little advancement. Low expectations and little variety. Generally low pay
Clubhouse work programmes	Jobs in-house, including clerical, maintenance and cooking	Meaningful work while feeling safe. Job belongs to clubhouse. No community integration. May not pay minimum wage
Community enterprises	E.g. bakery, cleaning company, convenience store, often part of clubhouse	Responsible work and a sense of belonging. Feels safe. Some community interaction but essentially an enclave. May not pay minimum wage
Transitional work programmes	Immediate placement into short-term entry level jobs, usually in the community. Accommodates special needs	Variety of jobs integrated into a community setting, but job does not belong to the person. May not pay minimum wage
Supported employment (SE)	Direct entry into competitive jobs with ongoing supports and clinical integration	Jobs belong to the person. Community integration. May take up to 6 months to find a suitable job. Minimum wage or better

as an evidence-based practice (Bond et al, 2001; Crowther et al, 2001). Most of these trials compared SE versus prevocational training or versus treatment as usual. Both types of employment service increased job tenure but people receiving SE were nearly three times more likely to be in employment at 12 months than people who had taken part in pre-vocational training (31 versus 12%), even when only the best quality trials were included (Crowther et al, 2001). People in SE also earned more and worked more hours than those who had received prevocational training. In addition, recent reports (Cook and Razzanno, 2000; Cook, 2001) from the Employment Intervention Demonstration Project (EIDP), a nationally funded evaluation of employment programmes for the mentally ill located in eight sites in the USA, found that partial employment in competitive work situations is possible for the majority of people with mental illness, particularly when SE principles are followed. After 6 months of receiving services, 40% of clients had obtained a job; after 12 months, 51% had obtained a job; by 24 months, 58% had obtained a job. Most of these jobs were low skilled and part-time, yet in normal work settings and at or above the minimum wage. After the first 6 months of service, 30–40% were generally employed at any one time. Of the various jobs obtained, 18% were full-time. These findings indicate that vocational rehabilitation can lead to improved work function, even if full-time work is not ultimately achieved.

The most clearly articulated and standardized approach to SE for people with severe mental illness is the individual placement and support (IPS) model (Drake and Becker, 1996). IPS has a number of critical elements that embody principles that aim to integrate vocational services with clinical care, providing optimal opportunities for community integration and personal independence (see Table 9.2).

The jobs in IPS may be opportunities that are specifically set aside for disabled people (available in some publicly funded organizations), or may be part-time jobs with significant accommodations (e.g. more frequent breaks, limited duties or greater tolerance for inconsistency). Nevertheless, these are jobs that clients can call their own and that pay a minimum wage or better. By offering jobs first, the IPS approach is in sharp contrast to rehabilitation programmes that offer skill training of

Table 9.2 Elements of Individual Placement and Support (IPS)

Elements	Comment
Commitment to competitive employment	Sometimes a brief trial period with an employer in which the client may be paid by the agency
Rapid job search	Clients find a job first and then are supported and trained as needed
Client preference essential	Client preferences, strengths and work experiences guide the job search
Commitment to the client and the employer	IPS job coaches make a commitment to the employer to stay involved indefinitely, offering support and assistance as needed
Integration between vocational services and mental health treatment	This is ideally achieved when IPS staff are actually a part of the treatment team

various kinds before placement in jobs. It is also strikingly different from programmes that offer graduated steps toward competitive employment. Finding employment may involve not only agency contacts but also personal connections through the client's family and friends. It is also recognized in IPS that the right fit between a person and the work environment is difficult to prejudge. Sometimes it is less the type of job than the qualities of the supervisor or the group of co-workers that makes for a good job fit. Trial and error is expected, with job loss seen as a necessary part of career development. On average, most workers in the general US population stay with their first job for less than 3 months, so IPS staff encourage their clients to keep trying until they find a job that suits them.

The indefinite commitment by IPS to the client and the employer can vary in intensity, with some impaired clients needing full-time coaching at the start and others needing only indirect assistance. Nevertheless, the episodic nature of mental illness and the difficulty clients may have with adapting to changes at work make it likely that many clients will have a crisis at work that requires a temporary intensification of supports. It is for this reason that follow-along services are so important for sustained competitive employment.

IPS also requires close integration between vocational services and mental health treatment. This integration is ideally achieved when IPS staff are a part of the treatment team. Assertive community treatment (ACT) programmes that offer ongoing integrated community mental health services have begun to include vocational services such as IPS in their treatment teams to good effect. In the USA, vocational services for the mentally ill are still much more likely to be contracted from providers who serve a wide range of handicapped clients. These providers are unaccustomed to the integration that IPS demands. Yet, clients are best served when all the professionals are working together toward the common goal of supporting that individual's highest level of function in the community. A simple example makes the point: a prescribing psychiatrist was unaware that their client had trouble staying awake at work because he was sedated after taking his afternoon medications. When informed of this problem by the job coach, the psychiatrist solved the problem by shifting the dosing schedule from three times daily to twice daily. Without integration, such an easily solved problem could become a reason for job failure.

These principles of IPS work best when used together and those programmes that are most faithful to the model generally have better outcomes (Bond et al, 2001a). To promulgate the use of supported employment, a Supported Employment Resource Kit (Becker, 2002) is being developed and will soon be available for distribution. It includes information and training materials for consumers, families, practitioners and administrators.

Conclusions

Work is important for recovery. Appropriate work, with proper support and accommodations, provides clinical benefits and community integration. As people with mental illness engage in productive roles and are empowered by their success, the general working population will get to know these individuals on a personal level. This will help society to understand mental illness better and may help reduce its terrible stigma.

References

Becker DR. *The Supported Employment Resource Kit.* (New Hampshire-Dartmouth Psychiatric Research Center: Concord, NH) (in press).

Bell M, Bryson G, Greig T et al. (2001) Neurocognitive enhancement therapy with work therapy. *Arch Gen Psychiatry*, **58:** 763–8.

Bell M, Lysaker P, Milstein R. (1996) Clinical benefits of paid work activity in schizophrenia. *Schizophrenia Bull*, **22:** 51–67.

Brigham A. (1847/1994) The moral treatment of insanity. *Am J Psychiatry*, **40:** 11–15.

Bryson GJ, Bell MD. (2002) Quality of life benefits of paid work activity. *Schizophrenia Bull*, **28:** 249–59.

Bond GR, Becker DR, Drake RE et al. (2001a) Implementing supported employment as an evidence-based practice. *Psychiatr Serv* **52:** 313–22.

Bond GR, Resnick SG, Drake RE et al. (2001b) Does competitive employment improve nonvocational outcomes for people with severe mental illness? *J Consult Clin Psychol* **6:** 489–501.

Cook J (2001). Early findings from the Employment Intervention Demonstration Program: what have we learned about innovative vocational models for people with psychiatric disability? Presented at the 26th Annual Conference of the International Association of Psychosocial Rehabilitation Services, Houston Texas.

Cook J, Razzanno L. (2000) Vocational rehabilitation for persons with schizophrenia: recent research and implications for practice. *Psychiatr Rehab J* **26:** 87–103.

Crowther R, Marshall M. (2001) Employment rehabilitation schemes for people with mental health problems in the North West region: service characteristics and utilisation. *J Ment Health* **10:** 373–81.

Crowther R, Marshall M, Bond G, Huxley P. (2001) Helping people with severe mental illness to obtain work: systematic review. *Br Med J* **322:** 204–8.

Drake RE, Becker DR. (1996) The individual placement and support model of supported employment. *Psychiatr Serv* **47:** 473–5.

McQuilken M, Zahniser JH, Novak J et al. (2002) The Work Project Survey: consumer perspectives on work. *J Vocat Rehab* (in press).

Mental Health Strategic Health Group (2001a) *Incentive Therapy FY 2001 Progress Report*. (Department of Veterans Affairs: Mental Health Strategic Health Group, Washington, DC.)

Mental Health Strategic Health Group (2001b) *Veterans Industries FY 2001 Progress Report*. (Department of Veterans Affairs: Washington, DC.)

Mueser KT, Becker DR, Torrey WC et al. (1997) Work and nonvocational domains of functioning in persons with severe mental illness: a longitudinal analysis. *J Nerv Ment Dis* **185**: 419–26.

National Institute of Disability and Rehabilitation Research (NIDRR) (1998) Strategies to secure and maintain employment for people with long-term mental illness. *Rehab Brief: Res Effect Focus* **15**: 1–4.

Priebe S, Warner R, Hubschmid T, Eckle I. (1998) Employment, attitudes toward work and quality of life among people with schizophrenia in three countries. *Schizophrenia Bull* **24**: 469–77.

Secker J, Grove B, Seebohm P. (2001) Challenging barriers to employment, training and education for mental health service users: the service user's perspective. *J Ment Health* **10**: 395–404.

Warr P. (1987) *Work, Unemployment and Mental Health* (Oxford University Press: Oxford.)

Whitaker R. (2002) *Mad in America*. (Perseus Publishing: Cambridge, MA.)

chapter 10

Family intervention in schizophrenia

Christine Barrowclough and Til Wykes

Families play an essential role in supporting people with long-term mental illness in the community. Over 60% of those with a first episode of a major mental illness return to live with relatives (Macmillan et al, 1986) and this appears to reduce only by 10–20% when those with subsequent admissions are included (Gibbons et al, 1984). However, the carer role is often not an easy one and may be associated with considerable personal costs. In schizophrenia, estimates from different studies suggest that up to two thirds of family members experience significant stress and subjective burden as a consequence of their caregiver role (Barrowclough et al, 1996). Not only is such stress likely to affect the well-being of the relatives and compromise their long-term ability to support the patient, but it may also have an impact on the course of the illness itself and on outcomes for the client. Hence, one of the most important advances in the treatment of schizophrenia in the last 20 years has been the development of family-based intervention programmes. The efficacy of this treatment is now well established, with many randomized controlled trials having demonstrated the superiority of family intervention over routine care in terms of patient relapse and hospitalization outcomes. This chapter outlines the background to this area of work, summarizes the research findings to date and draws attention to important areas for future development.

Background to family interventions in schizophrenia

The development of multifactorial models of the processes determining risk and relapse in schizophrenia provided the general rationale for the development of family interventions [see Clements and Turpin (1992) for a review of the models]. These stress–vulnerability models emphasized the contribution of psychological and socioenvironmental stressors to the illness course and thereby opened up the way to psychological interventions. In particular, family interventions found much of their initial impetus in the research on expressed emotion (EE). High EE is assessed on the basis of a critical, hostile or overinvolved attitude towards the patient on the part of a relative living in the same household. Early studies (Brown et al, 1972; Vaughn and Leff, 1976) found that when patients with schizophrenia were discharged home after being hospitalized for a relapse, their risk of subsequent relapse in the short term was greatly increased if at least one family member was assessed to be high EE. These results have been replicated many times and a meta-analysis of 27 studies (Butzlaff and Hooley, 1998) confirmed the elevated risk of relapse for patients in high EE households. So, within the context of stress–vulnerability models, an individual's home may be viewed as an environment capable of influencing the illness for better or worse. If attributes of certain households are responsible for precipitating relapse, then they might be identified and modified, with a resulting reduction in relapse rates. Throughout the past two decades a series of studies testing this theory have been reported and are described below.

Family-intervention studies

There have been several descriptive reviews of schizophrenia family-intervention studies (e.g. Barrowclough and Tarrier, 1984; Lam, 1991; Kavanagh, 1992; Dixon and Lehman, 1995; Penn and Mueser, 1996). Typically, the controlled trials recruited families at the point of hospitalization of a relative for an acute episode of schizophrenia and began the family intervention when the patient was discharged back to the home. The intervention period lasted from 6 to 12 months, at the end of which patient relapse rates were compared between those who received the family intervention as an adjunct to routine care and those who received routine care only. Routine care included the use of prophylactic medication.

A series of interventions were developed which differed in some important dimensions, including: the location of the family sessions (home versus hospital base); the number of sessions offered; the extent of the patient's involvement; the precise content of the sessions and the mode of delivery. Since there was no clear understanding of the mechanisms of patient relapse in the home environment, determining the content involved making assumptions about the kinds of problems associated with high EE families which might contribute to stress, and therefore the issues to be targeted. In practice, all the studies assumed that families had inadequate knowledge or misunderstandings regarding the illness and placed an emphasis on educating relatives about schizophrenia as an essential component, to the extent that some reviewers have subsumed all family intervention under the category psychoeducation. The other common strategy was helping the family members in coping with symptom-related difficulties either by a specific problem-solving approach (Falloon et al, 1982) or through assessment of individual problems and application of appropriate cognitive behavioural techniques (Barrowclough and Tarrier, 1992). Despite differences in approaches, Mari and Streiner (1994) have provided a useful summary of the common 'ingredients', or overall principles, of the treatments (see Box 10.1).

Results from the studies

A number of meta-analytic reviews of family-intervention studies have been published. These reviews include family-intervention studies where:

- the patient has a diagnosis of schizophrenia or schizoaffective disorder;

> ## Box 10.1 Common principles in successful family interventions.*
>
> To build up an alliance with relatives who care for the schizophrenic member
> To reduce adverse family atmosphere
> To enhance the problem-solving capacity of relatives
> To decrease expressions of anger and guilt
> To maintain reasonable expectations of patient performance
> To set limits safeguarding relatives' own well-being
> To achieve changes in relatives' behaviour and beliefs
>
> ---
>
> *From Mari and Streiner (1994).
> Reprinted with the permission of Cambridge University Press.

- there is some form of control or comparison group against which to evaluate any benefits from the experimental treatment;
- patient relapse or hospitalization is examined as the main outcome.

The analysis used by Pharoah et al (1999) adopted more stringent inclusion criteria and excluded studies if:

- there was non-random assignment;
- intervention was restricted to an inpatient intervention;
- the diagnosis was broader than schizophrenia;
- the intervention took place over fewer than five sessions.

Their review included 13 studies and concluded that family intervention as an adjunct to routine care decreased the frequency of relapse and hospitalization; these findings held across the wide age ranges, sex differences and variability in the length of illness found in the different studies. Moreover, the analysis suggested that these results generalize across care cultures where health systems are very different – trials from the UK, Australia, Europe, the People's Republic of China and the USA were included.

A more recent and inclusive review (Pitschel-Walz et al, 2001) examined 25 studies spanning 20 years (1977–1997) and again this meta-analysis confirmed the superiority of family-treated patient relapse rates over control groups, finding an effect size of 0.20, corresponding to a decrease in relapse rate of 20% in patients where families received an intervention. Although this treatment effect may seem relatively low, one must bear in mind that this analysis includes studies where the intervention was extremely brief and bore little resemblance to the intensive programmes in the original studies. For example, the studies of Falloon et al (1982), Leff et al (1982) and Tarrier et al (1988) (see Table 10.1) demonstrated decreased relapse rates for family-treated patients of around 40%. The absence of treatment fidelity measures in many of these studies makes it difficult to judge quality control within or between studies. Further comparison analyses within the review by Pitschel-Walz et al (2001) draw attention to some of the wide variations in the content and duration of programmes in recent years.

Longer term interventions were more successful than short-term interventions and more intensive family treatments were superior to a more limited approach (e.g. where relatives were offered little more than brief education sessions about schizophrenia). When families are provided with an 'effective dose' in terms of duration and intensity of intervention there is some evidence of the long-lasting effects from family treatment. Several studies (see Table 10.1) found a maintenance of the significant difference between the intervention and control groups at 2 years, and the 5- and 8-year follow-up data of Tarrier et al (1994) demonstrated how durable these effects can be. However, it must be emphasized that all the studies show that relapses increase with the number of years from termination of the intervention.

One of the criticisms of family-intervention studies has been their narrow focus on the end results of reductions in patient relapse and hospitalizations. The review by Pitschel-Walz et al (2001) suggests that there are some indications of family interventions having an impact over a wide range of outcomes, as shown in Table 10.1. For carers these include a reduction in carer burden, a change from high to low EE status and an improved knowledge about schizophrenia. For patients there is some evidence of better medication compliance [this effect would seem to be independent of the effect of family intervention (Hogarty et al, 1987; Sellwood et al, 2001)], improved quality of life and better social adjustment. Several studies have also demonstrated that these improved

Table 10.1 Controlled studies comparing family intervention with standard/alternative treatment for patients with schizophrenia (minimum 6 months intervention)

Study	Treatment conditions	No.	Type of family intervention	Duration of treatment	Relapse
Kottgen et al (1984)	(1) FI, high EE; (2) RC, high EE; (3) RC, low EE.	49	Psychodynamic groups	Up to 2 years	2 years: FI equal to RC for either high or low EE families
Falloon et al (1982, 1985)	(1) Behavioural FI + Individual patient treatment; (2) individual patient treatment	36	Home-based behavioural FI	2 years	2 years: behavioural FI superior to individual management
Leff et al (1982, 1985)	(1) FI; (2) RC	24	Groups + individual sessions; High EE learning from low EE	9 months	2 years: FI better than RC
Hogarty et al (1986, 1991)	(1) FI; (2) social skills; (3) combined FI + SS; (4) RC	180	Behavioural FI	Up to 2 years	2 years: FI better than RC or SS
Tarrier et al (1988,1989, 1994)	(1) Cognitive behavioural enactive and symbolic; (2) education only; (3) RC	83	Cognitive behavioural FI (families' choice of home or clinic)	9 months	2 years: FI better than education or RC; education and RC equal

Table 10.1 *continued*

Study	Treatment conditions	No.	Type of family intervention	Duration of treatment	Relapse
Leff et al (1990)	(1) Multiple-family psychoeducation and support; (2) single-family psychoeducation and support	23	Multiple-family groups in the clinic; single-family sessions at home	1 year	16 months: conditions equal
Mingyuan et al (1993)	(1) Mulitple-family psychoeducation and support; (2) RC	3092	Clinic-based lectures and discussions	1 year	1 year: multiple FI better than RC
Randolph et al (1994)	(1) Behavioural FI; (2) RC	39	Clinic-based behavioural FI	1 year	2 years: behavioural FI better than RC
Xiong et al (1994)	(1) Behavioural FI; (2) RC	63	Clinic-based psychoeducation, skills training, medication/ symptom management	18 months	18 months: behavioural FI better than RC
Zhang et al (1994)	(1) Multiple and single family; (2) psychoeducation and support	78	Multiple-family clinic-based psychoeducation counselling, medication/symptom management	1 year	18 months: family education and support better than RC

Table 10.1 continued

Study	Treatment conditions	No.	Type of family intervention	Duration of treatment	Relapse
Zastowny et al (1992)	(1) Behavioural FI; (2) Single-family psychoeducation and support	30	Hospital-based behavioural FI; hospital based single-family psychoeducational advice	1 year	16 months: conditions equal
McFarlane et al (1995)	(1) Multiple-family psychoeducation and support; (2) single-family psychoeducation and support	172	Multiple-family groups or single family sessions in the clinic	2 years	2 years: multiple-family conditions better than single-family condition
Linszen et al (1996)	(1) Behavioural FI + individual patient treatment; (2) Individual patient treatment	76	Hospital and home-based behavioural FI	1 year	1 year: conditions equal
Schooler et al (1997)	(1) Intensive behavioural FI; (2) supportive family management	313	Home-based behavioural FI plus supportive family management; supportive family management in clinic-based family groups	2 years	2 years: conditions equal

EE, Expressed emotion; FI, Family intervention; RC, Routine care; SS, Social skills training outcomes are achieved with reduced costs to society (e.g. Falloon et al, 1984; Tarrier, 1991; Xiong et al, 1994).

Dissemination of family interventions

In recent years there have been attempts to disseminate the benefits of family intervention in schizophrenia into routine service delivery. This has been largely through training programmes designed to provide clinicians, mainly community psychiatric nurses, with the knowledge and skills required to implement the family work [see Tarrier et al (1999) for a review of dissemination programmes]. Despite the solid evidence base for the efficacy of family-based psychological treatment programmes in schizophrenia, and the efforts of the training programmes, the implementation of family work in routine mental health services has been at best patchy. The consensus view in the literature is that family-intervention implementation faces complex organizational and attitudinal difficulties, and insufficient attention has been paid to these in dissemination programmes. In discussing the factors that might make the transfer from research to practice difficult, Mari and Streiner (1994) suggested that the requirements of durable-service-oriented interventions differ from those based on time-limited research models.

The need to change the clinical practice of the whole service, rather than simply training individuals, is underlined in the work of Corrigan and colleagues (Corrigan and McCracken, 1995a, b; Corrigan et al, 1997). However, difficulties arise not only from staff but also from carer reluctance to engage in family work. Several studies of community samples (e.g. McCreadie et al, 1991; Barrowclough et al, 1999) have shown that carer participation in family intervention is relatively low, with only around half of carers taking up the offer of either a support service or family intervention (Barrowclough et al, 1999), with possibly higher rates when help is offered at a time of crisis (Tarrier, 1991).

Summary and future directions

In summary, a number of important conclusions can be drawn from recent analyses of family-intervention studies. Firstly, whilst there is robust evidence for the efficacy of family interventions in schizophrenia, it is also clear that short education or counselling programmes do not affect relapse rates: 'a few lessons on schizophrenia . . . was simply not sufficient to substantially influence the relapse rate' (Pitschel-Walz et al, 2001, p. 84). The quality of interventions needs to be enhanced and monitored to ensure that families are offered the intensity of help likely to give them substantial benefits. Successful family interventions require considerable investment in time, skill and commitment; and since for many patients the effect is to delay rather than to prevent relapse, many patients and families will need long-term and continuing intervention. Work with relatives of recently diagnosed schizophrenia patients indicates that this help needs to begin from the first onset of the psychosis (Kuipers and Raune, 2000). Secondly, dissemination and engagement issues need to continue to be addressed. Although many patients and families benefit greatly from the intervention programmes, a substantial number of families are hard to engage and the implementation of family programmes within services presents many challenges. Finally, further work needs to be done to identify optimum techniques for changing family attitudes where problems are particularly complex, e.g. in schizophrenia and comorbid substance misuse (see also Chapter 6). The present authors are aware of only one recent trial that has evaluated a family-based component for this client group (Barrowclough et al, 2001).

References

Barrowclough C, Haddock G, Tarrier N et al. (2001) Randomised controlled trial of cognitive behavioral therapy plus motivational intervention for schizophrenia and substance use. *Am J Psychiatry* **158:** 1706–13.

Barrowclough C, Tarrier N. (1984) Psychosocial interventions with families and their effects on the course of schizophrenia: a review. *Psychol Med* **14:** 629–42.

Barrowclough C, Tarrier N. (1992) *Families of Schizophrenic Patients: Cognitive Behavioural Intervention.* (Chapman & Hall: London).

Barrowclough C, Tarrier N, Johnston M. (1996) Distress, expressed emotion and attributions in relatives of schizophrenic patients. *Schizophrenia Bull* 22: 691–701.

Barrowclough C, Tarrier N, Lewis S et al. (1999) Randomised controlled effectiveness trial of a needs–based psychosocial intervention service for carers of people with schizophrenia. *Br J Psychiatry* 174: 505–11.

Brown GW, Birley JLT, Wing JK. (1972) Influences of family life on the course of schizophrenic disorders: a replication. *Br J Psychiatry* 121: 241–8.

Butzlaff RL, Hooley JM. (1998) Expressed emotion and psychiatric relapse: a meta-analysis. *Arch Gen Psychiatry* 55: 547–52.

Clements K, Turpin G. (1992) *Innovations in the Psychological Management of Schizophrenia.* (John Wiley & Sons: Chichester).

Corrigan VA, McCracken SG. (1995a) Psychiatric rehabilitation and staff development: educational and organisational models. *Clin Psychol Rev* 15: 1172–7.

Corrigan VA, McCracken SG. (1995b) Refocusing the training of psychiatric rehabilitation staff. *Psychiatr Serv* 46: 1172–7.

Corrigan VA, McCracken SG, Edwards M et al. (1997) Collegial support and barriers to behavioural programs for severely mentally ill. *J Behav Ther Exp Psychiatry* 28: 193–202.

Dixon LB, Lehman AF. (1995) Family interventions for schizophrenia. *Schizophrenia Bull* 21: 631–43.

Falloon I, Boyd J, McGill C. (1984) *The Family of Care of Schizophrenia.* (Guilford: London).

Falloon IRH, Boyd JL, McGill CW et al. (1982) Family management in the prevention of exacerbations of schizophrenia. *N Engl J Med,* 306: 1437–40.

Falloon IRH, Boyd JL, McGill CW et al. (1985) Family management in the prevention of morbidity in schizophrenia: clinical outcome of a 2 year longitudinal study. *Arch Gen Psychiatry* 42: 887–96.

Gibbons JS, Horn SH, Powell JM et al. (1984) Schizophrenia patients and their families. A survey in a psychiatric service based on a district general hosptital. *Br J Psychiatry* 144: 70–7.

Hogarty G, Anderson CM, Reiss DJ et al. (1986) Family psychoeducation, social skills training and maintenance chemotherapy in the aftercare treatment of schizophrenia: one year effects of a controlled study on relapse and expressed emotion. *Arch Gen Psychiatry* 43: 633–42.

Hogarty G, Anderson CM, Reiss DJ. (1987) Family psychoeducation, social skills training and medication in schizophrenia: the long and the short of it. *Psychopharmacol Bull* 23: 12–13.

Hogarty G, Anderson CM, Reiss DJ et al. (1991) Family psychoeducation, social skills training and maintenance chemotherapy in the aftercare treatment of schizophrenia: two year effects of a controlled study on relapse and adjustment. *Arch Gen Psychitry* 48: 340–7.

Kavanagh D. (1992) Family interventions for schizophrenia. In: (Kavenagh DJ, ed) *Schizophrenia: An Overview and Practical Handbook.* (Chapman & Hall: London.)

Kottgen C, Soinnichesen I, Mollenhauer K, Jurth R. (1984) Results of the Hamburg Camberwell Family Interview Study, I-III. *Int J Family Psychiatry* 5: 61–94.

Kuipers E, Raune D. (2000) The early development of expressed emotion and burden in the families of first-onset psychosis. In: (Birchwood M, Fowler D, Jackson C, eds) *Early Intervention in Psychosis: A Guide to Concepts, Evidence & Interventions*. (John Wiley & Sons: Chichester.)

Lam DH. (1991) Psychosocial family intervention in schizophrenia: a review of empirical studies. *Psychol Med*, **21:** 423–41.

Leff JP, Berkowitz R, Shavit A et al. (1990) A trial of family therapy versus relatives' groups for schizophrenia. *Br J Psychiatry* **157:** 571–7.

Leff JP, Kuipers L, Berkowitz R et al. (1982) A controlled trial of intervention with families of schizophrenic patients. *Br J Psychiatry* **141:** 121–34.

Leff JP, Kuipers L, Sturgeon D. (1985) A controlled trial of social intervention in the families of schizophrenic patients. *Br J Psychiatry* **146:** 594–600.

Linszen D, Dingeman P, Van der Does JW et al. (1996) Treatment, expressed emotion and relapse in recent onset schizophrenia disorders. *Psychol Med* **26:** 333–42.

Macmillan JF, Gold A, Crow TJ et al. (1986) The Northwick Park Study of first episodes of schizophrenia: IV. Expressed emotion and relapse. *Br J Psychiatry* **148:** 133–43.

McCreadie RG, Phillips K, Harvey JA et al. (1991) The Nithscale schizophrenia surveys VIII. Do relatives want family intervention – and does it help? *Br J Psychiatry* **158:** 110–13.

McFarlane WR, Lukens E, Link B et al. (1995) Multiple family groups and psychoeducation in the treatment of schizophrenia. *Arch Gen Psychiatry* **52:** 679–87.

Mari JJ, Streiner DL. (1994) An overview of family interventions and relapse in schizophrenia: meta-analysis of research findings. *Psychol Med* **24:** 565–78.

Mari JJ, Streiner DL. (1996) Family intervention for people with schizophrenia (Cochrane Review). In: *The Cochrane Library*, Issue 1. (Update Software: Oxford, UK.)

Mingyuan Z, Heqin Y, Chengde Y et al. (1993) Effectiveness of psychoeducation of relatives of schizophrenic patients: a prospective cohort study in five cities of China. *Int J Ment Health* **22:** 47–59.

Penn DL, Mueser KT. (1996) Research update on the psychosocial treatment of schizophrenia. *Am J Psychiatry* **153:** 607–17.

Pharoah FM, Mari JJ, Streiner DL. (1999) Family intervention for people with schizophrenia (Cochrane Review) In: *The Cochrane Library*, Issue 4. (Update Software: Oxford, UK).

Pitschel-Walz G, Leucht S, Bauml J et al. (2001) The effect of family interventions on relapse and rehospitalisation in schizophrenia – a meta-analysis. *Schizophrenia Bull*, **27:** 73–92.

Randolph ET, Eth S, Glynn SM et al. (1994) Behavioural family management in schizophrenia: outcome of a clinic based intervention. *Br J Psychiatry* **164:** 501–6.

Schooler NR, Keith SJ, Severe JB et al. (1997) Relapse and rehospitalisation during maintenance treatment of schizophrenia. The effects of dose reduction and family treatment. *Arch Gen Psychiatry* **54:** 453–63.

Sellwood W, Barrowclough C, Tarrier N et al. (2001) Needs based cognitive behavioural family intervention for carers of patients suffering from schizophrenia: 12 month follow up. *Acta Psychiatr Scand* **104:** 346–55.

Tarrier N. (1991) Some aspects of family interventions in schizophrenia. I. Adherence with family intervention programmes. *Br J Psychiatry* **159**: 475–80.

Tarrier N, Lowson K, Barrowclough C. (1991) Some aspects of family interventions in schizophrenia. II: financial considerations. *Br J Psychiatry* **159**: 481–4.

Tarrier N, Barrowclough C, Haddock G, McGovern J. (1999) The dissemination of innovative cognitive–behavioural psychsocial treatments for schizophrenia. *J Ment Health* **8**: 569–82.

Tarrier N, Barrowclough C, Porceddu K, Fitzpatrick E. (1994) The Salford Family Intervention Project for schizophrenic relapse prevention: five and eight year accumulating relapses. *Br J Psychiatry* **165**: 829–32.

Tarrier N, Barrowclough C, Vaughn CE et al. (1989) The community management of schizophrenia: a controlled trial of a behavioural intervention with families to reduce relapse. *Br J Psychiatry* **153**: 532–42.

Vaughn C, Leff J. (1976) The influence of family and social factors on the course of psychiatric illness. *Br J Psychiatry* **129**: 125–37.

Xiong W, Phillips MR, Hu X et al. (1994) Family based intervention for schizophrenic patients in China: a randomised controlled trial. *Br J Psychiatry* **165**: 239–47.

Zastowny RR, Lehman AF, Cole RE, Kane C. (1992) Family management of schizophrenia: a comparison of behavioural and supportive family treatment. *Psychiatry Q,* **63**: 159–86.

Zhang M, Wang M, Li J, Phillips MR. (1994) Randomised control trial family intervention for 78 first episode male schizophrenic patients: an 18 month study in Suzhou, Japan. *Br J Psychiatry* **65** **(Suppl 24)**: 96–102.

Index

Note: Page references in *italics* refer to Figures; those in **bold** refer to Tables